COPD

DIET COOKBOOK

FOR BEGINNERS

Delicious and Nutritious Recipes to Breathe Easier, Boost Energy, and Improve Lung Health

Kingsley Klopp

Table of Contents

Poultry Recipes

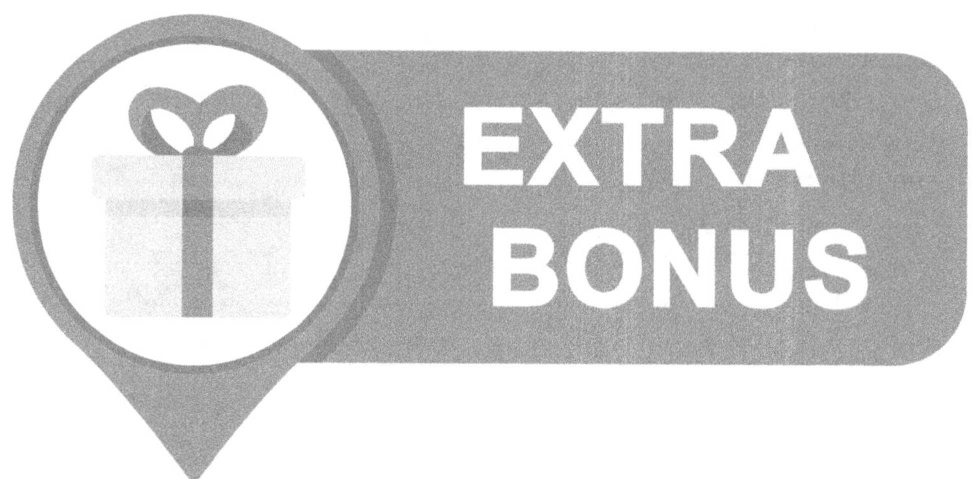

To show our appreciation for your purchase, we're delighted to offer you these special bonuses as a heartfelt thank you.

1. A Food Tracker Journal
2. Downloadable E-BOOK featuring full-color images of finished recipes

Important Note

We're thrilled to accompany you on this culinary journey towards better health and well-being. Before you dive into the delicious and nutritious recipes we've prepared, we want to share a gentle reminder to ensure your experience is both enjoyable and safe.

Every individual is unique, and so are their dietary needs. While our recipes are crafted to support those with COPD, it's important to remember that what works for one person may not work for another. Listen to your body and adjust the recipes according to your personal preferences and health requirements. If you have any specific dietary concerns or restrictions, we highly encourage you to consult with your healthcare provider or a registered dietitian. They can offer personalized advice and help you tailor the recipes to suit your needs.

Additionally, please keep in mind that the nutritional information provided in this cookbook is approximate. The values may vary depending on the specific ingredients you use and how you prepare the meals. While we've made every effort to ensure accuracy, slight variations are inevitable. Trust your instincts and, when in doubt, seek professional guidance.

We're here to inspire and guide you, but you know your body best. Make these recipes your own, and don't hesitate to reach out to your healthcare team if you have questions or concerns. Your well-being is our top priority, and we want you to feel confident and supported every step of the way.

Furthermore, If our cookbook has brought joy to your kitchen and table, we'd be thrilled to hear about your experiences in an Amazon review. On the flip side, if you stumble upon any hiccups while exploring our recipes, don't hesitate to get in touch at kloppkingsley@gmail.com. We're here to support your cooking journey every step of the way.

Happy cooking, and here's to a healthier, happier you!

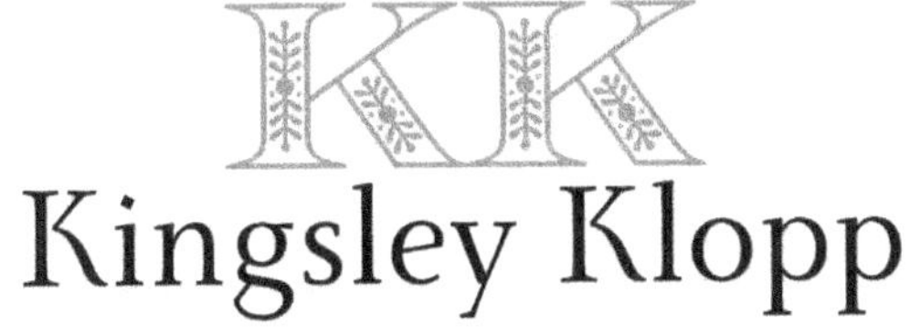

Kingsley Klopp

Introduction

Welcome to the **Chronic Obstructive Pulmonary Disease (COPD) Diet Cookbook for Beginners!** If you've picked up this book, you're likely on a journey to manage your COPD better, seeking ways to breathe easier, and live more comfortably. Whether you or a loved one has been recently diagnosed, or you've been managing COPD for years, this cookbook is designed to be a trusted companion in your kitchen, offering not just recipes but a pathway to improved health and well-being. Imagine waking up in the morning, feeling refreshed and ready to tackle the day. You head to the kitchen and whip up a delicious, nutritious breakfast that doesn't just fill your stomach but also supports your lungs. The recipes in this cookbook are crafted with love and expertise to help you achieve just that. Each dish is tailored to provide the nutrients needed to strengthen your respiratory system, reduce inflammation, and boost your overall health. And the best part? They are simple, easy-to-follow, and absolutely delicious. Living with COPD can sometimes feel like an uphill battle, but the good news is that the right diet can make a significant difference. Foods rich in antioxidants, vitamins, and healthy fats can play a crucial role in managing your symptoms and enhancing your quality of life. This cookbook demystifies the process of eating well with COPD. We'll walk you through the basics of nutrition, explain which foods are your best allies, and which ones to avoid, all while keeping the joy in cooking and eating.

You don't have to be a master chef to benefit from this book. Whether you're a novice in the kitchen or someone who enjoys cooking, you'll find these recipes approachable and rewarding. From hearty breakfasts to satisfying dinners, from savory snacks to delectable desserts, there's something here for every meal and every taste. Picture yourself savoring a flavorful bowl of chicken and vegetable soup on a chilly evening, or enjoying a refreshing fruit smoothie on a hot afternoon – all while knowing you're making choices that are good for your lungs. In addition to mouth-watering recipes, this cookbook also offers practical tips and strategies for meal planning and grocery shopping. We understand that living with COPD can sometimes limit your energy levels, so we've included time-saving tips and shortcuts to make meal preparation easier and more enjoyable. Plus, you'll find insights on how to maintain a balanced diet even on those tough days when cooking feels like a daunting task.

But this book isn't just about food – it's about empowerment. It's about taking control of your health and making choices that support your body's needs. It's about finding joy in nourishing yourself and discovering that eating well can be a delightful and empowering experience. By embracing the principles and recipes in this cookbook, you're taking a proactive step towards better health and a more vibrant life.

So, let's get cooking! With the **Chronic Obstructive Pulmonary Disease Diet Cookbook for Beginners** in your hands, you're equipped with the tools to make every meal a step towards better breathing and a happier, healthier you. Welcome to a journey of flavor, health, and vitality. Let's breathe easy and eat well together!

Chapter 1

UNDERSTANDING COPD.

When you or someone you love is diagnosed with Chronic Obstructive Pulmonary Disease (COPD), it can feel overwhelming. This chronic lung condition, which includes emphysema and chronic bronchitis, affects millions of people worldwide. It can make every breath feel like a struggle and turn everyday activities into daunting tasks. But understanding COPD is the first step towards managing it and reclaiming your life.

What is COPD?

COPD is a progressive lung disease characterized by increasing breathlessness. The airways in your lungs become inflamed and narrowed, and the air sacs lose their elasticity, making it hard for air to move in and out. This condition often develops from long-term exposure to irritants that damage your lungs, most commonly cigarette smoke. However, it can also be caused by environmental pollutants, genetic factors, and respiratory infections.

The Emotional Impact

Receiving a COPD diagnosis can be an emotional rollercoaster. You might feel fear, anger, sadness, or even a sense of loss. It's natural to mourn the activities you once enjoyed that now seem out of reach. But remember, while COPD changes your life, it doesn't define it. Embracing your emotions and seeking support from loved ones and healthcare professionals can make a significant difference in managing your condition.

Symptoms and Diagnosis of COPD

Chronic Obstructive Pulmonary Disease (COPD) is a long-term condition that makes breathing progressively more difficult. The journey with COPD often begins with subtle symptoms that are easy to dismiss but become increasingly severe over time. Understanding these symptoms and the diagnostic process is crucial for early intervention and better management of the disease.

Common Symptoms

1. **Chronic Cough:** One of the earliest and most persistent symptoms of COPD is a chronic cough, often referred to as a "smoker's cough." This cough is usually productive, meaning it brings up mucus (phlegm), and can be particularly bothersome in the morning.

2. **Shortness of Breath:** As the disease progresses, shortness of breath (dyspnea) becomes more noticeable. Initially, it might only occur during physical exertion, but over time, even simple tasks like walking or dressing can leave you breathless.

3. **Frequent Respiratory Infections:** People with COPD are more prone to respiratory infections, such as colds, flu, and pneumonia. These infections can exacerbate COPD symptoms and lead to further lung damage.

4. **Wheezing:** A whistling or squeaky sound when you breathe, known as wheezing, is another common symptom. It indicates that your airways are narrowed, making it difficult for air to move in and out.

5. **Chest Tightness:** Many people with COPD experience a feeling of tightness or heaviness in the chest. This sensation can be distressing and contribute to anxiety and discomfort.

6. **Fatigue:** Chronic fatigue is a frequent complaint among those with COPD. The effort of breathing, combined with poor oxygenation of the blood, can leave you feeling constantly tired and drained of energy.

Less Common Symptoms

- **Weight Loss:** In the later stages of COPD, weight loss and muscle wasting (cachexia) can occur, often due to the increased energy expenditure required for breathing.
- **Swelling in Ankles, Feet, or Legs:** This can be a sign of right-sided heart failure (cor pulmonale), a complication of severe COPD.

Diagnosis

Diagnosing COPD involves a combination of medical history, physical examinations, and specialized tests. Here's what you can expect during the diagnostic process:

1. **Medical History and Physical Exam:** Your doctor will ask about your symptoms, smoking history, exposure to lung irritants, and any family history of respiratory diseases. A physical exam will involve listening to your lungs with a stethoscope.
2. **Spirometry:** This is the most common and effective test for diagnosing COPD. Spirometry measures how much air you can exhale and how quickly, helping to identify airflow obstruction. During the test, you'll take a deep breath and blow into a tube connected to the spirometer.
3. **Chest X-ray or CT Scan:** Imaging tests like a chest X-ray or CT scan can provide a detailed view of your lungs and help identify any other conditions that might be causing your symptoms, such as lung cancer or infections.
4. **Arterial Blood Gas Analysis:** This test measures the levels of oxygen and carbon dioxide in your blood, giving insight into how well your lungs are functioning.
5. **Other Lung Function Tests:** Additional tests, such as a lung diffusion capacity test or plethysmography, may be used to assess the severity of your lung impairment.

Key Nutrients for Lung Health.

1. Omega-3 Fatty Acids

Omega-3 fatty acids, found in fish such as salmon, mackerel, and sardines, as well as in flaxseeds and walnuts, have potent anti-inflammatory properties. Chronic inflammation is a significant factor in COPD, and omega-3s can help reduce this inflammation, improving lung function and reducing symptoms. Including these fatty acids in your diet can help mitigate the inflammatory processes that damage lung tissues over time.

2. Antioxidants

Antioxidants play a vital role in protecting the lungs from oxidative stress and damage caused by free radicals. Vitamins C and E are powerful antioxidants. Vitamin C, found in citrus fruits, strawberries, bell peppers, and broccoli, helps boost the immune system and protect the lungs from infections. Vitamin E, found in nuts, seeds, and green leafy vegetables, supports lung health by preventing oxidative damage to lung tissues.

3. Vitamin D

Vitamin D is essential for immune function and has been shown to reduce the risk of respiratory infections. Sun exposure is a primary source of vitamin D, but it can also be obtained from foods like fortified dairy products, fatty fish, and egg yolks. Adequate levels of vitamin D can help maintain healthy lung function and reduce the severity of COPD symptoms.

4. Magnesium

Magnesium is a mineral that plays a crucial role in lung function. It helps relax the bronchial muscles, making it easier to breathe. Foods rich in magnesium include spinach, nuts, seeds, and whole grains. Ensuring sufficient magnesium intake can help manage symptoms like wheezing and shortness of breath.

5. Zinc

Zinc is vital for maintaining a healthy immune system and aiding in the repair of damaged tissues. It can help reduce the frequency and severity of respiratory infections, which are common in COPD patients. Foods high in zinc include meat, shellfish, legumes, and seeds.

6. Vitamin A

Vitamin A is essential for maintaining the health of the mucous membranes lining the respiratory tract. This vitamin can be found in foods like carrots, sweet potatoes, and dark leafy greens. It helps keep these membranes healthy, reducing the risk of infections and supporting overall lung function.

7. Selenium

Selenium is a trace mineral with antioxidant properties that protect lung tissues from oxidative damage. It also plays a role in preventing infections and reducing inflammation. Brazil nuts, seafood, and whole grains are excellent sources of selenium.

8. Protein

Protein is crucial for maintaining and repairing body tissues, including the lungs. Individuals with COPD often experience muscle wasting, and adequate protein intake can help prevent this. Lean meats, poultry, fish, eggs, dairy products, legumes, and nuts are good sources of protein.

9. Fiber

Dietary fiber, found in fruits, vegetables, whole grains, and legumes, supports overall health, including lung health. A high-fiber diet can improve cardiovascular health, which is closely linked to respiratory health, and reduce the risk of conditions that can exacerbate COPD.

Incorporating these key nutrients into your diet can significantly impact lung health, especially for those managing COPD. A balanced diet rich in omega-3 fatty acids, antioxidants, vitamins, minerals, protein, and fiber can help reduce inflammation, boost the immune system, and support overall respiratory function. Remember, making informed dietary choices is a proactive step towards better lung health and improved quality of life.

Foods to Include and Avoid

Foods to Include

1. **Fruits and Vegetables**: Fresh fruits and vegetables are rich in vitamins, minerals, and antioxidants that help reduce inflammation and protect lung tissues. Berries, oranges, apples, tomatoes, leafy greens, and cruciferous vegetables like broccoli and cauliflower are particularly beneficial. They provide essential nutrients like vitamins C and E, beta-carotene, and potassium, which support immune function and lung health.

2. **Omega-3 Fatty Acids**: Found in fatty fish like salmon, mackerel, and sardines, as well as in flaxseeds, chia seeds, and walnuts, omega-3 fatty acids have powerful anti-inflammatory properties. Including these foods in your diet can help reduce lung inflammation and improve overall respiratory function.

3. **Whole Grains**: Whole grains like oats, brown rice, quinoa, and whole wheat products provide fiber, vitamins, and minerals that support cardiovascular health, which is closely linked to lung health. A diet rich in whole grains can help manage blood pressure and reduce the risk of comorbid conditions that can worsen COPD symptoms.

4. **Lean Proteins**: Protein is essential for maintaining muscle strength, including the respiratory muscles. Lean meats, poultry, fish, eggs, legumes, and low-fat dairy products are excellent sources of protein. Adequate protein intake can help prevent muscle wasting and maintain respiratory function.

5. **Nuts and Seeds**: Nuts and seeds are rich in healthy fats, protein, magnesium, and other essential nutrients. They can provide a quick energy boost and are easy to incorporate into meals and snacks. Almonds, sunflower seeds, and pumpkin seeds are particularly good choices.

6. **Hydrating Fluids**: Staying well-hydrated is crucial for thinning mucus, making it easier to expel. Water, herbal teas, and broths are excellent hydrating fluids. Avoid sugary drinks and opt for hydration options that support overall health.

Foods to Avoid

1. **Processed Foods**: Processed foods, including fast food, snacks, and pre-packaged meals, are often high in salt, sugar, and unhealthy fats. These ingredients can exacerbate inflammation, increase blood pressure, and lead to weight gain, all of which can negatively impact lung health.

2. **High-Sodium Foods**: Excessive sodium intake can lead to fluid retention and increase the workload on the heart and lungs. Avoiding foods high in sodium, such as canned soups, processed meats, and salty snacks, can help manage symptoms. Opt for low-sodium alternatives and season foods with herbs and spices instead of salt.

3. Sugary Foods and Beverages: High sugar intake can lead to weight gain and increased inflammation. Sugary foods and beverages, such as candies, pastries, sodas, and sweetened juices, should be limited. Choose naturally sweet options like fruits or small amounts of dark chocolate for a healthier alternative.

4. Dairy Products: Some individuals with COPD find that dairy products can thicken mucus, making it harder to clear. While dairy is a good source of calcium and vitamin D, if you notice increased mucus production after consuming dairy, consider reducing your intake or switching to plant-based alternatives like almond milk or soy yogurt.

4. Fried and Greasy Foods: Fried and greasy foods can cause bloating and discomfort, making breathing more difficult. Foods like french fries, fried chicken, and greasy burgers should be avoided. Instead, choose baked, grilled, or steamed options.

5. Carbonated Beverages: Carbonated drinks can cause bloating and gas, which can put extra pressure on the diaphragm and make breathing more difficult. Avoid sodas and sparkling waters, and stick to still water and non-carbonated beverages.

Breakfast Recipes

1. Oatmeal with Honey
Ingredients:
- 1 cup rolled oats
- 2 cups water or milk (dairy or non-dairy)
- 1 tablespoon honey
- 1/2 teaspoon cinnamon
- 1/4 teaspoon vanilla extract
- 1/4 cup fresh berries (blueberries, strawberries, or raspberries)
- 1 tablespoon chopped nuts (almonds, walnuts, or pecans)

Instructions:
1. In a medium saucepan, bring the water or milk to a boil.
2. Add the rolled oats and reduce the heat to a simmer. Cook for 5-7 minutes, stirring occasionally, until the oats are tender and the liquid is absorbed.
3. Remove from heat and stir in the honey, cinnamon, and vanilla extract.
4. Top with fresh berries and chopped nuts.
5. Serve warm.

Nutrition Info (per serving):
- Calories: 250
- Protein: 7g
- Carbohydrates: 40g
- Fiber: 6g
- Sugars: 12g
- Fat: 8g
- Sodium: 30mg

Number of Servings: 2
Cooking Time: 10 minutes

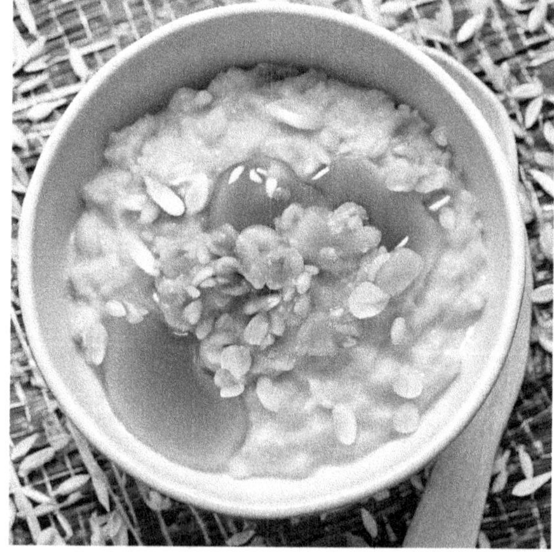

2. Egg and Avocado Bowl

Ingredients:

- 2 large eggs
- 1 ripe avocado
- 1/4 teaspoon paprika
- 1 tablespoon lemon juice
- 1/4 cup cherry tomatoes, halved
- 1 tablespoon chopped fresh parsley
- 1 slice whole-grain toast

Instructions:

1. Bring a small pot of water to a boil and gently lower the eggs into the pot. Cook for 8-10 minutes for hard-boiled eggs.
2. While the eggs are cooking, cut the avocado in half, remove the pit, and scoop the flesh into a bowl. Mash with a fork and mix in the lemon juice and paprika.
3. Toast the slice of whole-grain bread.
4. Once the eggs are done, peel and slice them.
5. Spread the mashed avocado on the toast, top with sliced eggs, cherry tomatoes, and chopped parsley.
6. Serve immediately.

Nutrition Info (per serving):

- Calories: 350
- Protein: 14g
- Carbohydrates: 26g
- Fiber: 10g
- Sugars: 3g
- Fat: 24g
- Sodium: 220mg

Number of Servings: 1
Cooking Time: 15 minutes

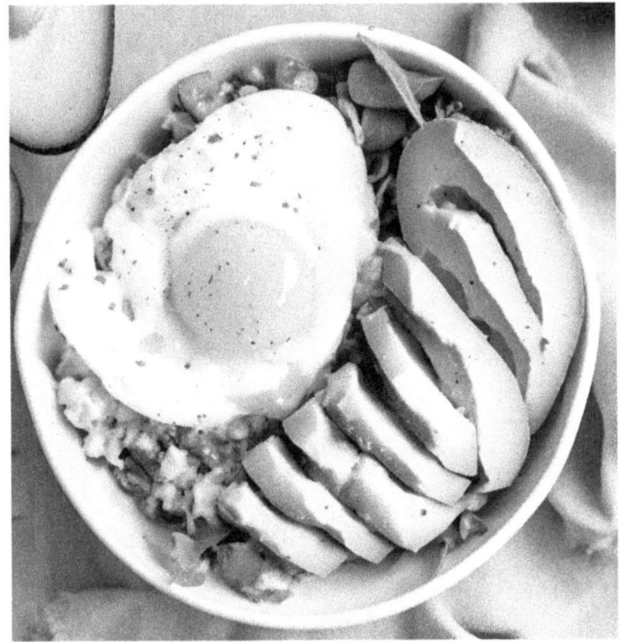

3. Buckwheat Porridge with Almonds

Ingredients:

- 1 cup buckwheat groats
- 2 cups water
- 1 cup almond milk (or other non-dairy milk)
- 1 tablespoon maple syrup
- 1/4 cup chopped almonds
- 1/4 teaspoon cinnamon
- 1/4 teaspoon nutmeg
- 1/4 cup dried fruit (raisins, cranberries, or apricots)

Instructions:

1. Rinse the buckwheat groats under cold water.
2. In a medium saucepan, combine the buckwheat groats, water, and almond milk. Bring to a boil over medium-high heat.
3. Reduce the heat to low and simmer for 15 minutes, stirring occasionally, until the buckwheat is tender and the liquid is absorbed.
4. Stir in the maple syrup, cinnamon, nutmeg, chopped almonds, and dried fruit.
5. Serve warm.

Nutrition Info (per serving):

- Calories: 320
- Protein: 9g
- Carbohydrates: 53g
- Fiber: 8g
- Sugars: 12g
- Fat: 10g
- Sodium: 50mg

Number of Servings: 2
Cooking Time: 20 minutes

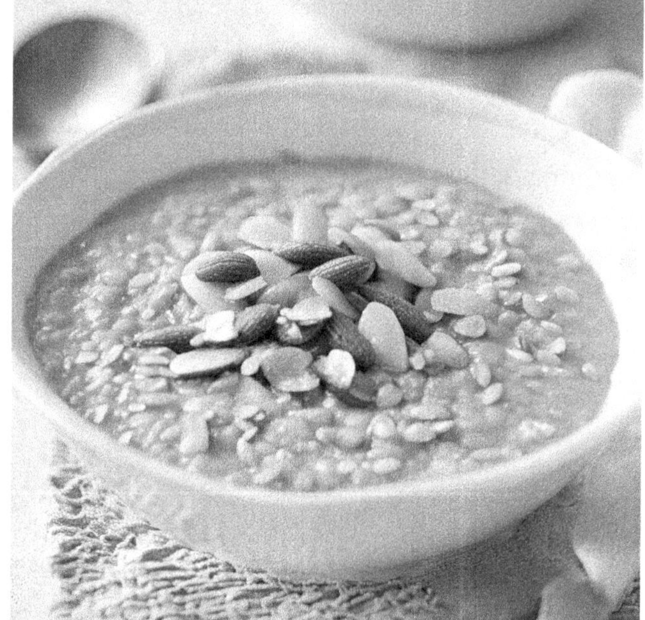

4. Protein-Packed Pancakes

Ingredients:

- 1 cup whole wheat flour
- 1 scoop protein powder (vanilla or unflavored)
- 1 teaspoon baking powder
- 1/2 teaspoon baking soda
- 1 teaspoon cinnamon
- 1 cup unsweetened almond milk
- 1 large egg
- 1 tablespoon honey
- 1 teaspoon vanilla extract
- 1/4 cup Greek yogurt
- 1/4 cup fresh berries (optional, for topping)

Instructions:

1. In a large bowl, whisk together the flour, protein powder, baking powder, baking soda, and cinnamon.
2. In another bowl, whisk together the almond milk, egg, honey, and vanilla extract.
3. Pour the wet ingredients into the dry ingredients and mix until just combined.
4. Heat a non-stick skillet or griddle over medium heat and lightly grease it with cooking spray or a small amount of oil.
5. Pour 1/4 cup of batter onto the skillet for each pancake. Cook until bubbles form on the surface, then flip and cook until golden brown, about 2-3 minutes per side.
6. Serve the pancakes topped with Greek yogurt and fresh berries.

Nutrition Info (per serving):

- Calories: 290
- Protein: 18g
- Carbohydrates: 40g
- Fiber: 6g
- Sugars: 10g
- Fat: 7g
- Sodium: 300mg

Number of Servings: 3
Cooking Time: 20 minutes

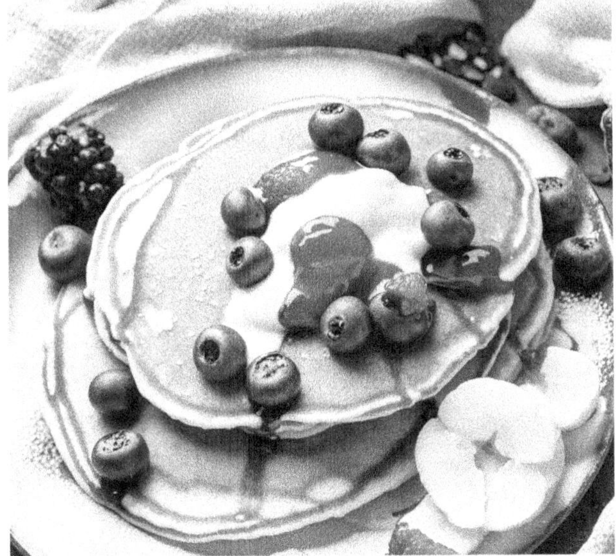

5. Savory Muffins with Veggies

Ingredients:

- 1 cup whole wheat flour
- 1/2 cup almond flour
- 1 teaspoon baking powder
- 1/2 teaspoon baking soda
- 1/4 teaspoon turmeric
- 1/4 teaspoon cumin
- 1/4 teaspoon garlic powder
- 1/2 cup grated zucchini
- 1/2 cup grated carrot
- 1/4 cup chopped spinach
- 1/4 cup chopped red bell pepper
- 1/2 cup unsweetened almond milk
- 1/4 cup olive oil
- 2 large eggs
- 1/4 cup grated Parmesan cheese

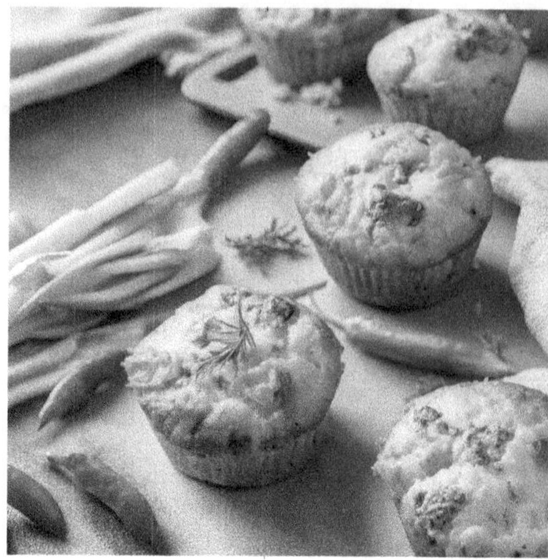

Instructions:

1. Preheat the oven to 350°F (175°C) and line a muffin tin with paper liners or lightly grease it.
2. In a large bowl, whisk together the whole wheat flour, almond flour, baking powder, baking soda, turmeric, cumin, and garlic powder.
3. In another bowl, whisk together the almond milk, olive oil, and eggs.
4. Pour the wet ingredients into the dry ingredients and mix until just combined.
5. Fold in the grated zucchini, grated carrot, chopped spinach, and chopped red bell pepper.
6. Spoon the batter into the muffin tin, filling each cup about 2/3 full.
7. Sprinkle the tops with grated Parmesan cheese.
8. Bake for 20-25 minutes, or until a toothpick inserted into the center of a muffin comes out clean.
9. Allow the muffins to cool in the tin for 5 minutes before transferring them to a wire rack to cool completely.

Nutrition Info (per serving):

- Calories: 180
- Protein: 5g
- Carbohydrates: 14g
- Fiber: 3g
- Sugars: 3g
- Fat: 11g
- Sodium: 150mg

Number of Servings: 12 muffins

Cooking Time: 30 minutes

6. Herbed Cream Cheese on Bagel

Ingredients:
- 1 whole-grain bagel
- 4 oz (113g) low-fat cream cheese
- 1 tablespoon chopped fresh chives
- 1 tablespoon chopped fresh parsley
- 1 teaspoon lemon zest
- 1/4 teaspoon garlic powder
- 1/4 teaspoon paprika
- 1/2 cup sliced cucumber

Instructions:
1. In a small bowl, mix the cream cheese, chives, parsley, lemon zest, garlic powder, and paprika until well combined.
2. Toast the whole-grain bagel.
3. Spread the herbed cream cheese on the toasted bagel halves.
4. Top with sliced cucumber.
5. Serve immediately.

Nutrition Info (per serving):
- Calories: 320
- Protein: 12g
- Carbohydrates: 45g
- Fiber: 5g
- Sugars: 8g
- Fat: 10g
- Sodium: 400mg

Number of Servings: 2
Cooking Time: 10 minutes

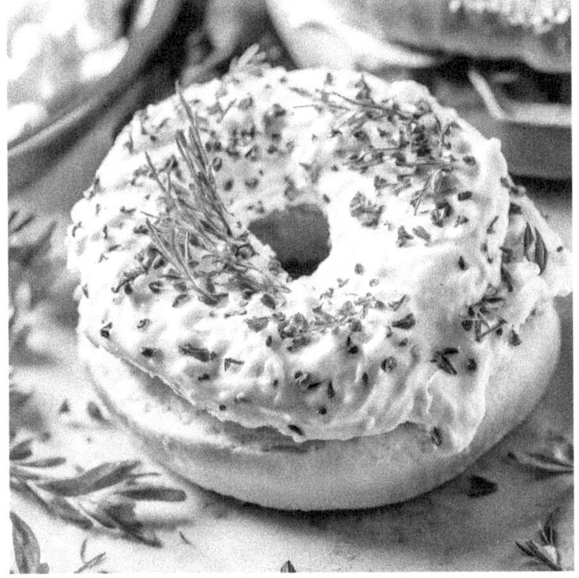

7. Pineapple Cottage Cheese

Ingredients:

- 1 cup low-fat cottage cheese
- 1 cup fresh pineapple chunks
- 1 tablespoon chia seeds
- 1/4 teaspoon cinnamon
- 1 tablespoon honey

Instructions:

1. In a bowl, combine the cottage cheese and fresh pineapple chunks.
2. Sprinkle with chia seeds and cinnamon.
3. Drizzle with honey.
4. Mix gently and serve.

Nutrition Info (per serving):

- Calories: 200
- Protein: 14g
- Carbohydrates: 28g
- Fiber: 4g
- Sugars: 18g
- Fat: 4g
- Sodium: 400mg

Number of Servings: 2
Cooking Time: 5 minutes

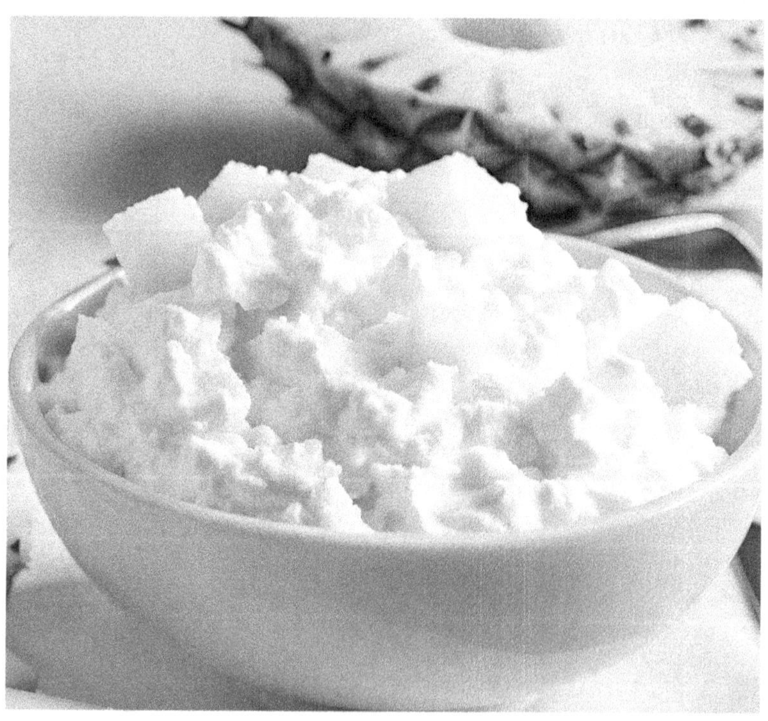

8. Spinach and Feta Wrap

Ingredients:

- 1 whole-grain tortilla
- 1 cup fresh spinach leaves
- 1/4 cup crumbled feta cheese
- 1 large egg
- 1 tablespoon olive oil
- 1/4 teaspoon dried oregano
- 1/4 teaspoon garlic powder
- 1/4 cup cherry tomatoes, halved

Instructions:

1. Heat the olive oil in a non-stick skillet over medium heat.
2. Add the spinach and cook until wilted, about 2-3 minutes.
3. In a bowl, whisk the egg with oregano and garlic powder.
4. Pour the egg mixture into the skillet with the spinach and cook until the egg is fully set, about 3-4 minutes.
5. Remove from heat and let it cool slightly.
6. Place the tortilla on a flat surface. Add the spinach and egg mixture, crumbled feta cheese, and cherry tomatoes.
7. Roll up the tortilla and cut in half.
8. Serve warm.

Nutrition Info (per serving):

- Calories: 350
- Protein: 15g
- Carbohydrates: 32g
- Fiber: 6g
- Sugars: 4g
- Fat: 18g
- Sodium: 550mg

Number of Servings: 1
Cooking Time: 10 minutes

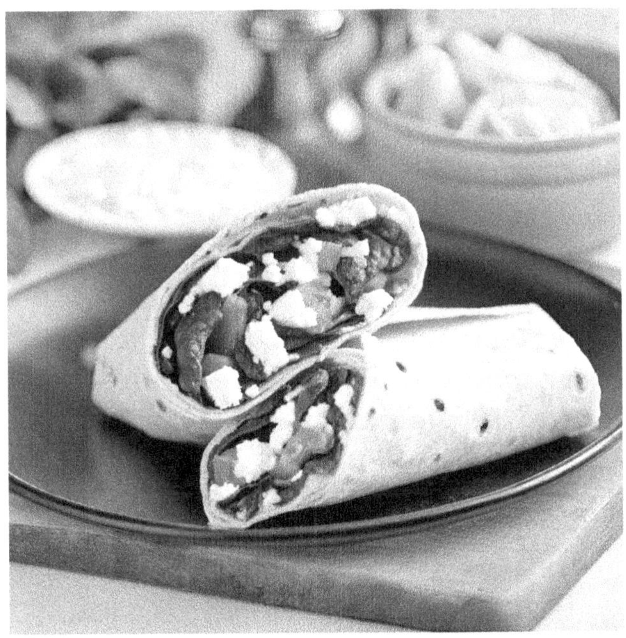

9. Spiced Pear Baked Oatmeal

Ingredients:

- 1 cup rolled oats
- 2 cups almond milk
- 1 large pear, diced
- 1/4 cup chopped walnuts
- 1/4 cup maple syrup
- 1 teaspoon cinnamon
- 1/2 teaspoon ground ginger
- 1/4 teaspoon ground nutmeg
- 1 teaspoon vanilla extract
- 1/2 teaspoon baking powder

Instructions:

1. Preheat the oven to 350°F (175°C) and lightly grease an 8x8-inch baking dish.
2. In a large bowl, mix the rolled oats, baking powder, cinnamon, ground ginger, and nutmeg.
3. In another bowl, whisk together the almond milk, maple syrup, and vanilla extract.
4. Pour the wet ingredients into the dry ingredients and mix until combined.
5. Fold in the diced pear and chopped walnuts.
6. Pour the mixture into the prepared baking dish.
7. Bake for 30-35 minutes, or until the top is golden brown and the oatmeal is set.
8. Let cool for a few minutes before serving.

Nutrition Info (per serving):

- Calories: 270
- Protein: 5g
- Carbohydrates: 45g
- Fiber: 6g
- Sugars: 20g
- Fat: 9g
- Sodium: 60mg

Number of Servings: 4
Cooking Time: 40 minutes

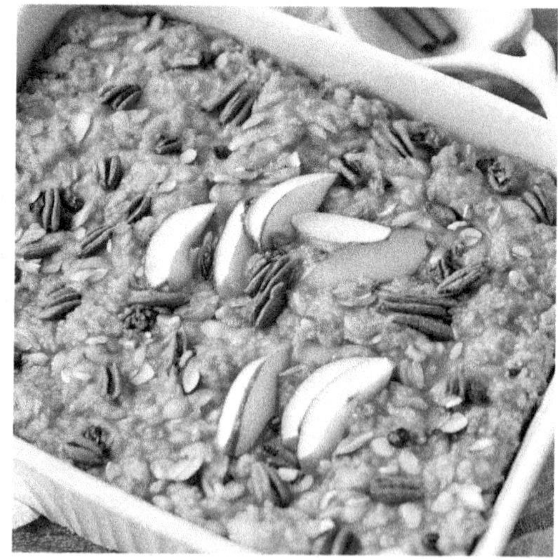

10. Fruit and Nut Yogurt
Ingredients:

- 1 cup Greek yogurt
- 1/2 cup mixed fresh fruit (such as berries, diced apples, or sliced bananas)
- 2 tablespoons chopped nuts (almonds, walnuts, or pecans)
- 1 tablespoon honey
- 1 teaspoon chia seeds

Instructions:

1. Spoon the Greek yogurt into a bowl.
2. Top with mixed fresh fruit.
3. Sprinkle with chopped nuts and chia seeds.
4. Drizzle with honey.
5. Serve immediately.

Nutrition Info (per serving):

- Calories: 250
- Protein: 12g
- Carbohydrates: 30g
- Fiber: 5g
- Sugars: 18g
- Fat: 10g
- Sodium: 80mg

Number of Servings: 1
Cooking Time: 5 minutes

11. Vegetable Hash

Ingredients:

- 1 medium sweet potato, peeled and diced
- 1 small red bell pepper, diced
- 1 small zucchini, diced
- 1/2 small red onion, diced
- 2 tablespoons olive oil
- 1 teaspoon paprika
- 1/4 teaspoon turmeric
- 1/4 teaspoon cumin
- 2 large eggs
- 1 tablespoon chopped fresh parsley

Instructions:

1. Heat 1 tablespoon of olive oil in a large skillet over medium heat.
2. Add the diced sweet potato and cook for 5-7 minutes, until slightly tender.
3. Add the bell pepper, zucchini, and red onion to the skillet. Cook for another 5-7 minutes, stirring occasionally, until the vegetables are tender.
4. Add the paprika, turmeric, and cumin. Stir to combine and cook for another 2 minutes.
5. In a separate small skillet, heat the remaining tablespoon of olive oil over medium heat.
6. Crack the eggs into the skillet and cook until the whites are set but the yolks are still runny, about 3-4 minutes.
7. Divide the vegetable hash between two plates and top each with a cooked egg.
8. Sprinkle with chopped fresh parsley and serve immediately.

Nutrition Info (per serving):

- Calories: 300
- Protein: 10g
- Carbohydrates: 35g
- Fiber: 8g
- Sugars: 12g
- Fat: 15g
- Sodium: 120mg

Number of Servings: 2
Cooking Time: 20 minutes

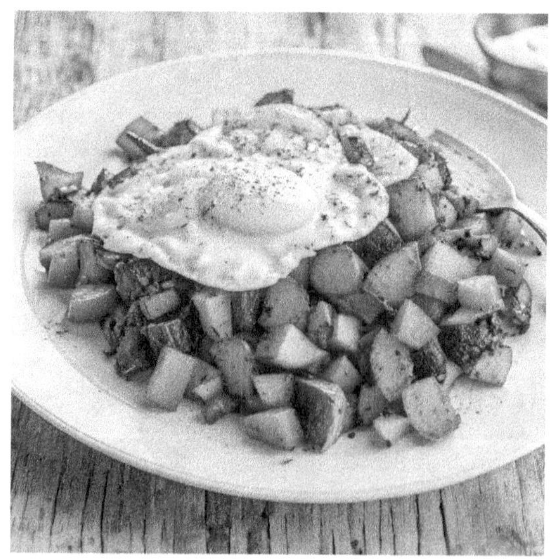

12. Banana Nut Waffles

Ingredients:

- 1 cup whole wheat flour
- 1/4 cup chopped walnuts
- 1 teaspoon baking powder
- 1/2 teaspoon baking soda
- 1 teaspoon cinnamon
- 1 large ripe banana, mashed
- 1 cup almond milk
- 1 large egg
- 1 tablespoon honey
- 1 teaspoon vanilla extract

Instructions:

1. Preheat your waffle iron according to the manufacturer's instructions.
2. In a large bowl, whisk together the flour, chopped walnuts, baking powder, baking soda, and cinnamon.
3. In another bowl, whisk together the mashed banana, almond milk, egg, honey, and vanilla extract.
4. Pour the wet ingredients into the dry ingredients and mix until just combined.
5. Lightly grease the waffle iron and pour the batter into the waffle iron, cooking according to the manufacturer's instructions until the waffles are golden brown and crisp.
6. Serve warm with additional banana slices and chopped walnuts if desired.

Nutrition Info (per serving):

- Calories: 280
- Protein: 8g
- Carbohydrates: 42g
- Fiber: 5g
- Sugars: 12g
- Fat: 10g
- Sodium: 300mg

Number of Servings: 4
Cooking Time: 15 minutes

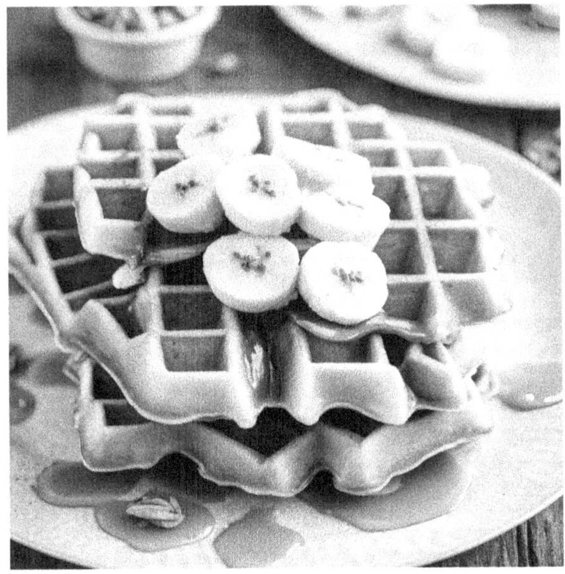

13. Smoked Salmon on Rye
Ingredients:
- 2 slices rye bread
- 4 oz (113g) smoked salmon
- 2 tablespoons low-fat cream cheese
- 1 tablespoon chopped fresh dill
- 1 teaspoon lemon juice
- 1/4 teaspoon garlic powder
- 1/4 cup sliced cucumber
- 1/4 cup sliced red onion

Instructions:
1. Toast the rye bread slices.
2. In a small bowl, mix the cream cheese, chopped dill, lemon juice, and garlic powder until well combined.
3. Spread the herbed cream cheese mixture on the toasted rye bread slices.
4. Top with smoked salmon, sliced cucumber, and sliced red onion.
5. Serve immediately.

Nutrition Info (per serving):
- Calories: 290
- Protein: 16g
- Carbohydrates: 24g
- Fiber: 4g
- Sugars: 4g
- Fat: 14g
- Sodium: 600mg

Number of Servings: 2
Cooking Time: 10 minutes

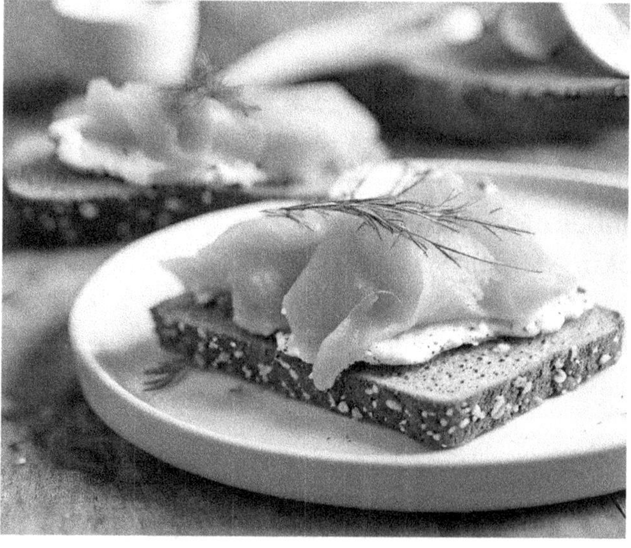

14. Zucchini Bread
Ingredients:

- 1 1/2 cups whole wheat flour
- 1 teaspoon baking powder
- 1/2 teaspoon baking soda
- 1 teaspoon cinnamon
- 1/2 teaspoon nutmeg
- 1/4 teaspoon ginger powder
- 1/2 cup unsweetened applesauce
- 1/2 cup honey
- 2 large eggs
- 1 teaspoon vanilla extract
- 1 1/2 cups grated zucchini
- 1/2 cup chopped walnuts (optional)

Instructions:

1. Preheat the oven to 350°F (175°C). Grease and flour a 9x5-inch loaf pan.
2. In a large bowl, whisk together the flour, baking powder, baking soda, cinnamon, nutmeg, and ginger powder.
3. In another bowl, mix the applesauce, honey, eggs, and vanilla extract until well combined.
4. Add the wet ingredients to the dry ingredients and stir until just combined.
5. Fold in the grated zucchini and chopped walnuts, if using.
6. Pour the batter into the prepared loaf pan and spread evenly.
7. Bake for 50-60 minutes, or until a toothpick inserted into the center comes out clean.
8. Allow to cool in the pan for 10 minutes, then transfer to a wire rack to cool completely before slicing.

Nutrition Info (per serving):

- Calories: 200
- Protein: 4g
- Carbohydrates: 30g
- Fiber: 3g
- Sugars: 18g
- Fat: 7g
- Sodium: 120mg

Number of Servings: 10
Cooking Time: 60 minutes

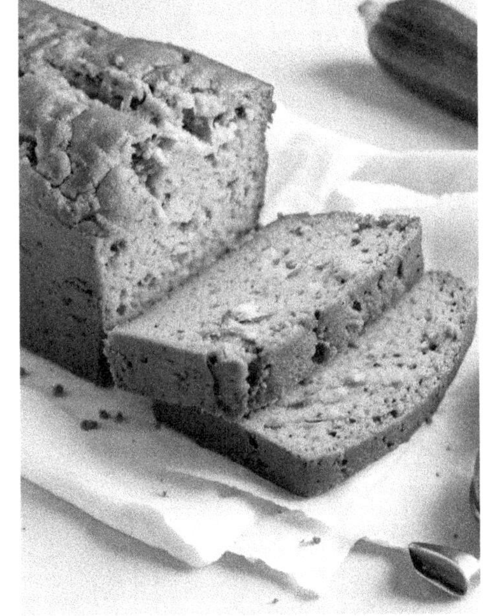

15. Barley and Mushroom Breakfast Bowl

Ingredients:

- 1 cup pearl barley
- 2 1/2 cups vegetable broth
- 1 tablespoon olive oil
- 1 cup sliced mushrooms (any variety)
- 1/2 cup diced onion
- 1 clove garlic, minced
- 1 tablespoon chopped fresh parsley
- 1 teaspoon thyme
- 1/4 cup grated Parmesan cheese

Instructions:

1. Rinse the barley under cold water. In a medium saucepan, bring the vegetable broth to a boil.
2. Add the barley, reduce the heat, and simmer for 30-40 minutes, or until tender and the liquid is absorbed.
3. While the barley is cooking, heat the olive oil in a large skillet over medium heat. Add the onions and cook until translucent, about 5 minutes.
4. Add the sliced mushrooms and garlic to the skillet and cook until the mushrooms are tender, about 5-7 minutes.
5. Stir in the thyme and parsley, and cook for another 2 minutes.
6. Once the barley is cooked, add it to the skillet with the mushroom mixture and stir to combine.
7. Serve topped with grated Parmesan cheese.

Nutrition Info (per serving):

- Calories: 250
- Protein: 7g
- Carbohydrates: 45g
- Fiber: 8g
- Sugars: 4g
- Fat: 7g
- Sodium: 350mg

Number of Servings: 4
Cooking Time: 45 minutes

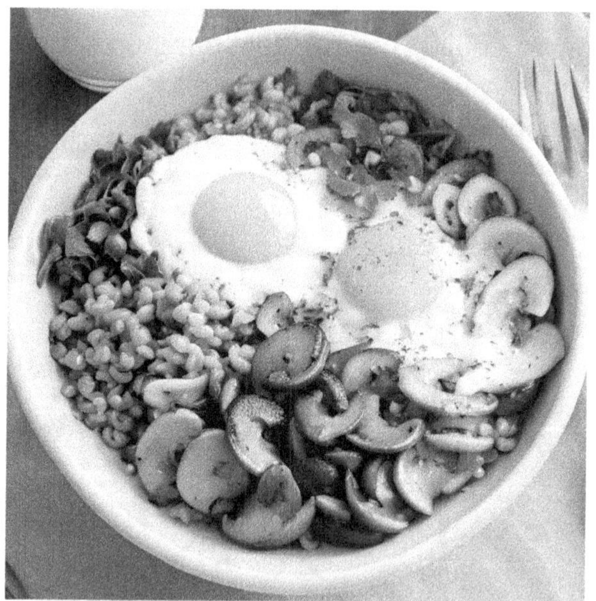

16. Peach Ricotta Crepes

Ingredients:

- 1 cup whole wheat flour
- 1 1/2 cups almond milk
- 2 large eggs
- 1 tablespoon honey
- 1 teaspoon vanilla extract
- 1/2 cup ricotta cheese
- 2 peaches, sliced
- 1 tablespoon maple syrup
- 1/4 teaspoon cinnamon

Instructions:

1. In a bowl, whisk together the flour, almond milk, eggs, honey, and vanilla extract until smooth.
2. Heat a non-stick skillet over medium heat and lightly grease it with cooking spray or a small amount of oil.
3. Pour 1/4 cup of batter into the skillet and swirl to spread evenly. Cook for 2-3 minutes until the edges start to lift, then flip and cook for another 1-2 minutes. Repeat with the remaining batter.
4. In another bowl, mix the ricotta cheese with maple syrup and cinnamon.
5. Spread a tablespoon of the ricotta mixture onto each crepe and top with sliced peaches.
6. Roll up the crepes and serve warm.

Nutrition Info (per serving):

- Calories: 200
- Protein: 9g
- Carbohydrates: 32g
- Fiber: 4g
- Sugars: 15g
- Fat: 6g
- Sodium: 100mg

Number of Servings: 6
Cooking Time: 20 minutes

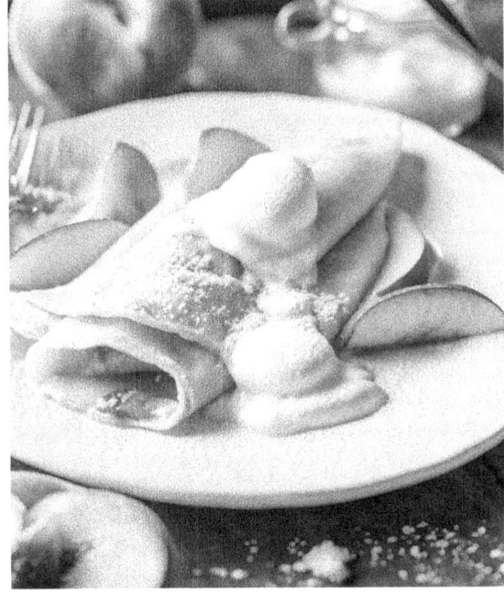

17. Vegetable Omelet

Ingredients:

- 2 large eggs
- 1/4 cup diced bell peppers (any color)
- 1/4 cup diced tomatoes
- 1/4 cup chopped spinach
- 1/4 cup diced mushrooms
- 1 tablespoon olive oil
- 1/4 teaspoon garlic powder
- 1 tablespoon chopped fresh basil

Instructions:

1. Heat the olive oil in a non-stick skillet over medium heat.
2. Add the bell peppers, tomatoes, spinach, and mushrooms. Cook for 3-5 minutes until the vegetables are tender.
3. In a bowl, whisk the eggs with the garlic powder.
4. Pour the eggs over the vegetables in the skillet and cook until the eggs are set, about 3-4 minutes.
5. Sprinkle with chopped fresh basil and fold the omelet in half.
6. Serve warm.

Nutrition Info (per serving):

- Calories: 220
- Protein: 12g
- Carbohydrates: 6g
- Fiber: 2g
- Sugars: 3g
- Fat: 16g
- Sodium: 140mg

Number of Servings: 1
Cooking Time: 10 minutes

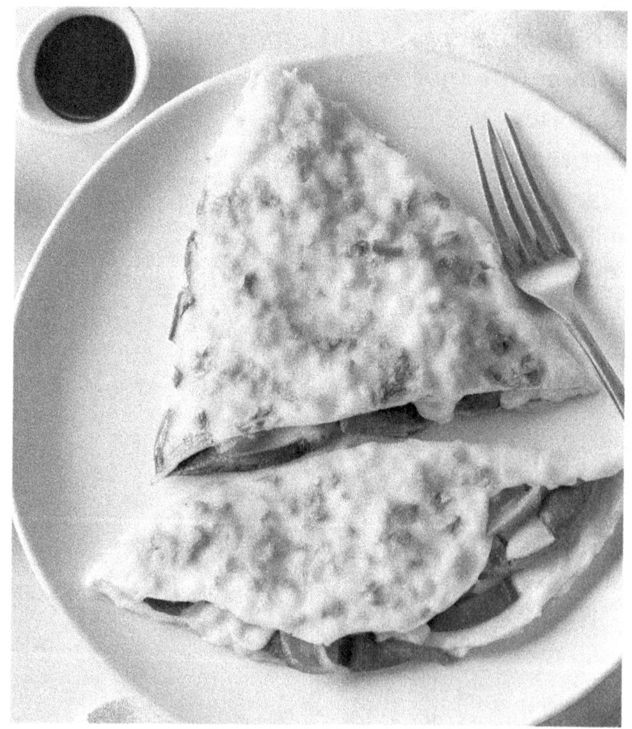

18. Baked Apple Oatmeal

Ingredients:

- 1 1/2 cups rolled oats
- 2 cups almond milk
- 2 apples, diced
- 1/4 cup maple syrup
- 1 teaspoon cinnamon
- 1/2 teaspoon nutmeg
- 1/4 teaspoon ground cloves
- 1 teaspoon vanilla extract
- 1/4 cup chopped pecans

Instructions:

1. Preheat the oven to 350°F (175°C). Grease an 8x8-inch baking dish.
2. In a large bowl, mix the rolled oats, almond milk, diced apples, maple syrup, cinnamon, nutmeg, cloves, and vanilla extract until well combined.
3. Pour the mixture into the prepared baking dish and spread evenly.
4. Sprinkle the chopped pecans on top.
5. Bake for 30-35 minutes, or until the top is golden brown and the oatmeal is set.
6. Let cool for a few minutes before serving.

Nutrition Info (per serving):

- Calories: 220
- Protein: 5g
- Carbohydrates: 38g
- Fiber: 5g
- Sugars: 16g
- Fat: 6g
- Sodium: 60mg

Number of Servings: 6
Cooking Time: 35 minutes

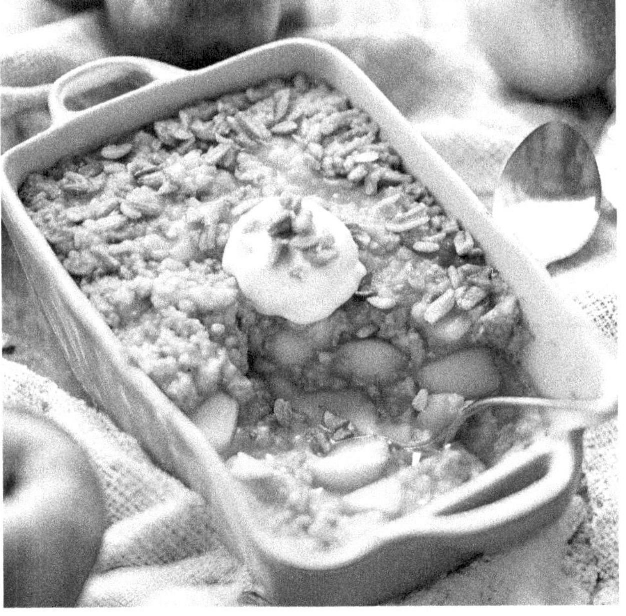

19. Quinoa Fruit Salad

Ingredients:

- 1 cup cooked quinoa
- 1 cup mixed fresh fruit (such as berries, diced apples, or sliced bananas)
- 1/4 cup chopped nuts (almonds, walnuts, or pecans)
- 1 tablespoon honey
- 1 tablespoon lemon juice
- 1 teaspoon chia seeds

Instructions:

1. In a large bowl, combine the cooked quinoa and mixed fresh fruit.
2. In a small bowl, whisk together the honey and lemon juice.
3. Pour the honey and lemon juice mixture over the quinoa and fruit, and toss to combine.
4. Sprinkle with chopped nuts and chia seeds.
5. Serve immediately.

Nutrition Info (per serving):

- Calories: 220
- Protein: 5g
- Carbohydrates: 40g
- Fiber: 6g
- Sugars: 14g
- Fat: 7g
- Sodium: 20mg

Number of Servings: 4

Cooking Time: 10 minutes

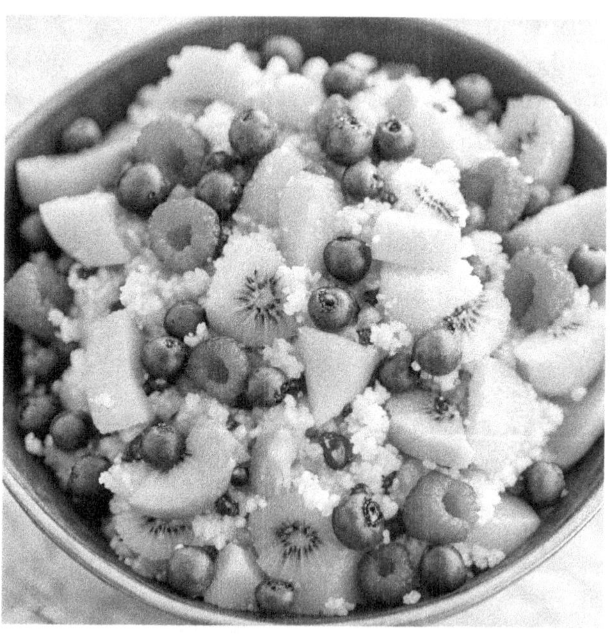

20. Pumpkin Pancakes

Ingredients:

- 1 cup whole wheat flour
- 1 teaspoon baking powder
- 1/2 teaspoon baking soda
- 1 teaspoon cinnamon
- 1/2 teaspoon nutmeg
- 1/4 teaspoon ground ginger
- 1/2 cup pumpkin puree
- 1 cup almond milk
- 1 large egg
- 2 tablespoons honey
- 1 teaspoon vanilla extract

Instructions:

1. In a large bowl, whisk together the flour, baking powder, baking soda, cinnamon, nutmeg, and ginger.
2. In another bowl, whisk together the pumpkin puree, almond milk, egg, honey, and vanilla extract.
3. Pour the wet ingredients into the dry ingredients and mix until just combined.
4. Heat a non-stick skillet or griddle over medium heat and lightly grease it with cooking spray or a small amount of oil.
5. Pour 1/4 cup of batter onto the skillet for each pancake. Cook until bubbles form on the surface, then flip and cook until golden brown, about 2-3 minutes per side.
6. Serve warm with maple syrup or your favorite pancake toppings.

Nutrition Info (per serving):

- Calories: 180
- Protein: 5g
- Carbohydrates: 30g
- Fiber: 4g
- Sugars: 10g
- Fat: 4g
- Sodium: 200mg

Number of Servings: 4

Cooking Time: 15 minutes

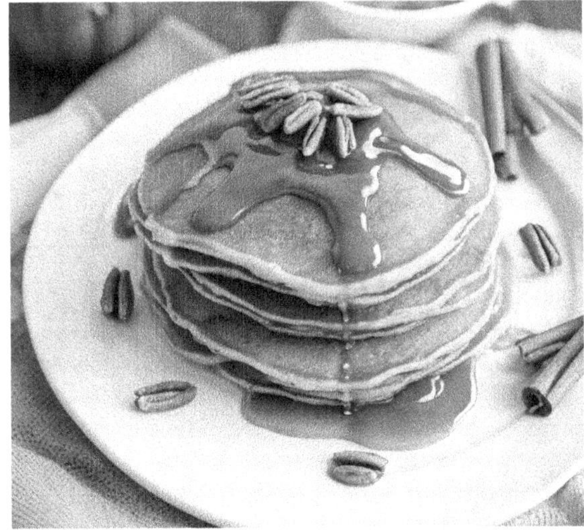

21. Almond Butter Banana Smoothie

Ingredients:

- 1 large ripe banana
- 1 cup almond milk
- 2 tablespoons almond butter
- 1 tablespoon honey
- 1/4 teaspoon cinnamon
- 1/2 teaspoon vanilla extract
- 1 cup ice cubes

Instructions:

1. In a blender, combine the banana, almond milk, almond butter, honey, cinnamon, vanilla extract, and ice cubes.
2. Blend until smooth and creamy.
3. Pour into glasses and serve immediately.

Nutrition Info (per serving):

- Calories: 280
- Protein: 5g
- Carbohydrates: 35g
- Fiber: 5g
- Sugars: 22g
- Fat: 14g
- Sodium: 80mg

Number of Servings: 2
Cooking Time: 5 minutes

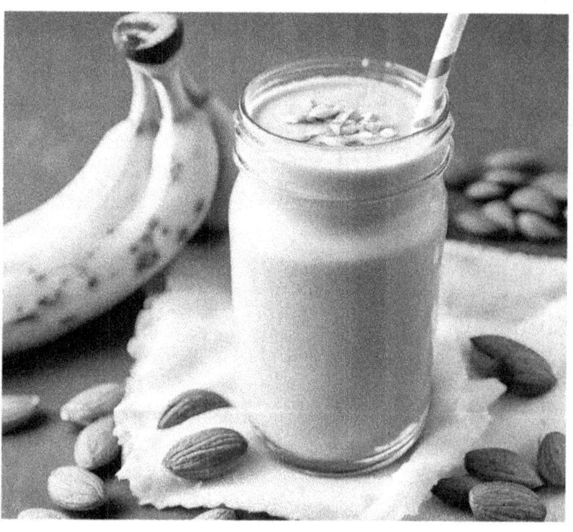

22. Apple Cinnamon Porridge

Ingredients:

- 1 cup rolled oats
- 2 cups almond milk
- 1 apple, diced
- 1 tablespoon honey
- 1 teaspoon cinnamon
- 1/4 teaspoon nutmeg
- 1/4 cup chopped walnuts

Instructions:

1. In a medium saucepan, bring the almond milk to a boil.
2. Add the rolled oats and reduce the heat to a simmer. Cook for 5-7 minutes, stirring occasionally, until the oats are tender and the liquid is absorbed.
3. Stir in the diced apple, honey, cinnamon, and nutmeg. Cook for another 2-3 minutes until the apple is tender.
4. Remove from heat and top with chopped walnuts.
5. Serve warm.

Nutrition Info (per serving):

- Calories: 250
- Protein: 6g
- Carbohydrates: 40g
- Fiber: 6g
- Sugars: 18g
- Fat: 8g
- Sodium: 40mg

Number of Servings: 2
Cooking Time: 10 minutes

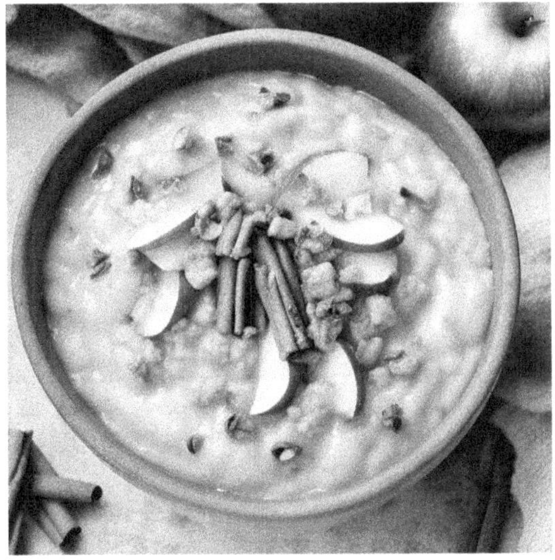

Fish & Seafood Recipes

1. Grilled Salmon with Lemon and Dill
Ingredients:
- 4 salmon fillets (about 6 oz each)
- 2 tablespoons olive oil
- 2 tablespoons fresh lemon juice
- 2 teaspoons lemon zest
- 2 tablespoons chopped fresh dill
- 1 garlic clove, minced

Instructions:
1. Preheat the grill to medium-high heat.
2. In a small bowl, mix the olive oil, lemon juice, lemon zest, chopped dill, and minced garlic.
3. Brush the salmon fillets with the lemon and dill mixture.
4. Place the salmon fillets on the grill, skin-side down, and cook for 4-5 minutes per side, or until the salmon is cooked through and flakes easily with a fork.
5. Remove from the grill and serve immediately.

Nutrition Info (per serving):
- Calories: 350
- Protein: 34g
- Carbohydrates: 1g
- Fiber: 0g
- Sugars: 0g
- Fat: 22g
- Sodium: 80mg

Number of Servings: 4
Cooking Time: 10 minutes

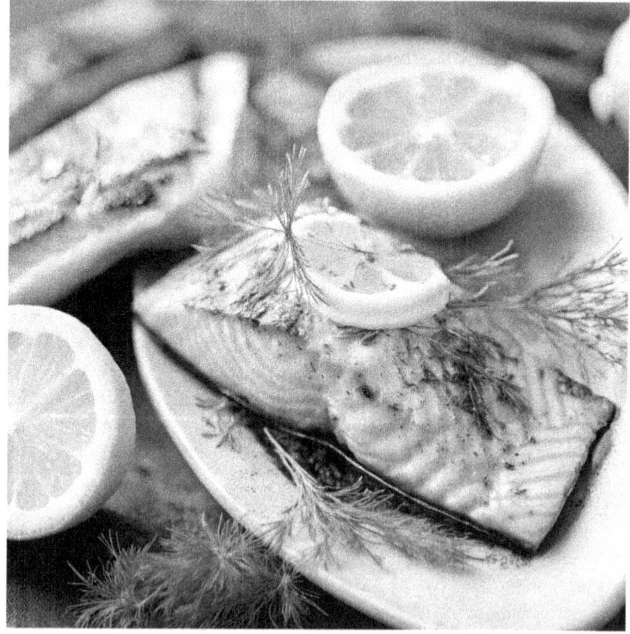

2. Shrimp Stir-Fry

Ingredients:

- 1 lb large shrimp, peeled and deveined
- 2 tablespoons olive oil
- 1 red bell pepper, sliced
- 1 yellow bell pepper, sliced
- 1 cup snap peas
- 1 cup broccoli florets
- 3 garlic cloves, minced
- 1 tablespoon grated ginger
- 2 tablespoons low-sodium soy sauce
- 1 tablespoon sesame oil
- 1 teaspoon honey
- 1 tablespoon chopped fresh cilantro

Instructions:

1. Heat the olive oil in a large skillet or wok over medium-high heat.
2. Add the garlic and ginger, and cook for 1-2 minutes until fragrant.
3. Add the shrimp to the skillet and cook until they turn pink and are cooked through, about 3-4 minutes. Remove the shrimp and set aside.
4. In the same skillet, add the bell peppers, snap peas, and broccoli. Stir-fry for 5-6 minutes until the vegetables are tender-crisp.
5. Return the shrimp to the skillet.
6. In a small bowl, mix the soy sauce, sesame oil, and honey. Pour over the shrimp and vegetables, stirring to coat evenly.
7. Cook for an additional 2-3 minutes until heated through.
8. Sprinkle with chopped fresh cilantro and serve immediately.

Nutrition Info (per serving):

- Calories: 250
- Protein: 24g
- Carbohydrates: 12g
- Fiber: 3g
- Sugars: 6g
- Fat: 11g
- Sodium: 500mg

Number of Servings: 4
Cooking Time: 15 minutes

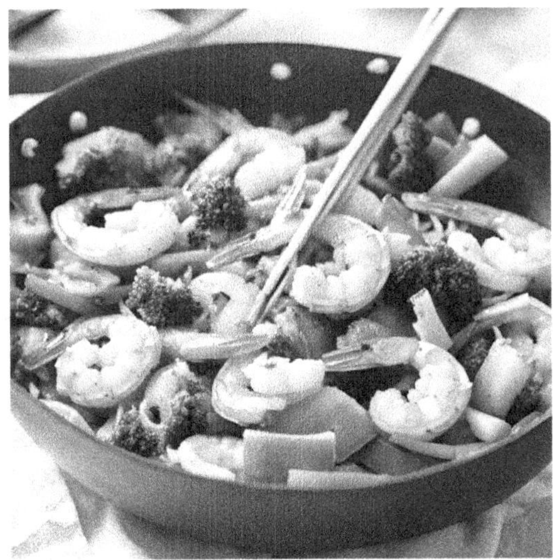

3. Mackerel Salad

Ingredients:

- 2 smoked mackerel fillets
- 4 cups mixed salad greens
- 1 cup cherry tomatoes, halved
- 1/2 cucumber, sliced
- 1/4 red onion, thinly sliced
- 1 avocado, sliced
- 2 tablespoons olive oil
- 1 tablespoon lemon juice
- 1 teaspoon Dijon mustard
- 1/2 teaspoon honey
- 1 tablespoon chopped fresh parsley

Instructions:

1. In a large bowl, combine the mixed salad greens, cherry tomatoes, cucumber, red onion, and avocado.
2. Flake the smoked mackerel fillets into bite-sized pieces and add to the salad.
3. In a small bowl, whisk together the olive oil, lemon juice, Dijon mustard, and honey.
4. Drizzle the dressing over the salad and toss gently to combine.
5. Sprinkle with chopped fresh parsley and serve immediately.

Nutrition Info (per serving):

- Calories: 350
- Protein: 18g
- Carbohydrates: 12g
- Fiber: 6g
- Sugars: 6g
- Fat: 26g
- Sodium: 400mg

Number of Servings: 2
Cooking Time: 10 minutes

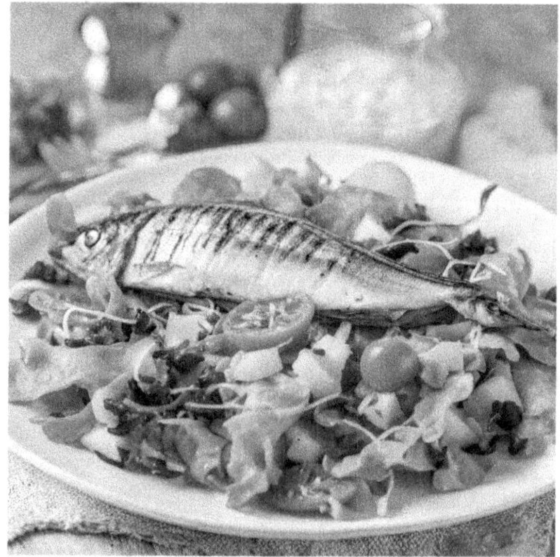

4. Garlic Butter Scallops

Ingredients:

- 1 lb large sea scallops
- 2 tablespoons unsalted butter
- 3 garlic cloves, minced
- 1 tablespoon olive oil
- 1 tablespoon lemon juice
- 1 teaspoon lemon zest
- 2 tablespoons chopped fresh parsley

Instructions:

1. Pat the scallops dry with a paper towel.
2. Heat the olive oil in a large skillet over medium-high heat.
3. Add the scallops to the skillet and cook for 2-3 minutes on each side until golden brown and cooked through. Remove the scallops from the skillet and set aside.
4. In the same skillet, add the butter and minced garlic. Cook for 1-2 minutes until the garlic is fragrant.
5. Stir in the lemon juice and lemon zest.
6. Return the scallops to the skillet and toss to coat in the garlic butter sauce.
7. Sprinkle with chopped fresh parsley and serve immediately.

Nutrition Info (per serving):

- Calories: 250
- Protein: 20g
- Carbohydrates: 4g
- Fiber: 0g
- Sugars: 0g
- Fat: 18g
- Sodium: 450mg

Number of Servings: 4
Cooking Time: 10 minutes

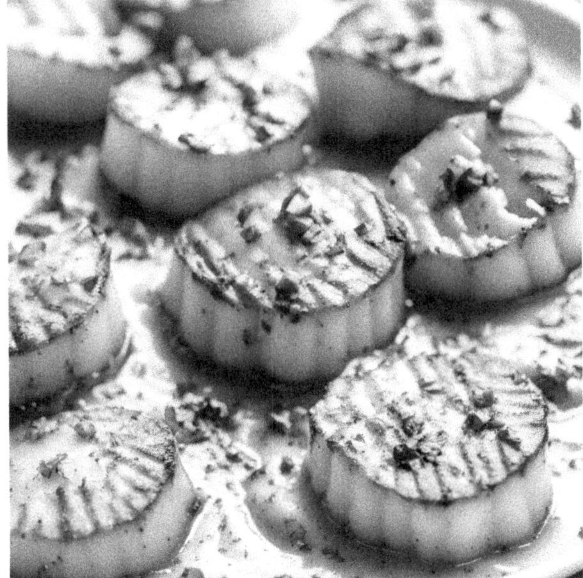

5. Linguine with Clam Sauce

Ingredients:

- 8 oz whole wheat linguine
- 2 tablespoons olive oil
- 3 garlic cloves, minced
- 1/2 cup dry white wine
- 2 cans (6.5 oz each) chopped clams, with juice
- 1/2 teaspoon red pepper flakes
- 1 tablespoon lemon juice
- 1 teaspoon lemon zest
- 1/4 cup chopped fresh parsley

Instructions:

1. Cook the linguine according to the package instructions until al dente. Drain and set aside.
2. Heat the olive oil in a large skillet over medium heat.
3. Add the minced garlic and red pepper flakes to the skillet and cook for 1-2 minutes until fragrant.
4. Pour in the white wine and cook for 2-3 minutes until the liquid is reduced by half.
5. Add the chopped clams with their juice to the skillet and stir to combine.
6. Stir in the lemon juice and lemon zest.
7. Add the cooked linguine to the skillet and toss to coat in the sauce.
8. Sprinkle with chopped fresh parsley and serve immediately.

Nutrition Info (per serving):

- Calories: 350
- Protein: 20g
- Carbohydrates: 45g
- Fiber: 6g
- Sugars: 2g
- Fat: 10g
- Sodium: 600mg

Number of Servings: 4

Cooking Time: 20 minute

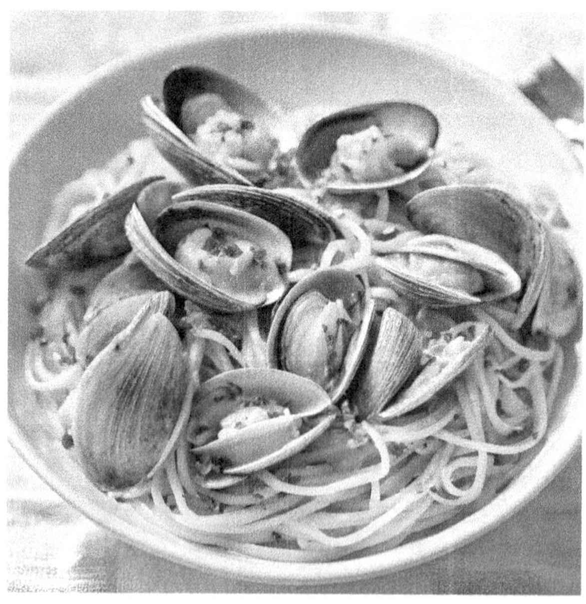

6. Baked Haddock with Olives and Capers

Ingredients:

- 4 haddock fillets (about 6 oz each)
- 2 tablespoons olive oil
- 1/2 cup sliced green olives
- 2 tablespoons capers, rinsed
- 1 lemon, thinly sliced
- 2 garlic cloves, minced
- 1 tablespoon fresh parsley, chopped
- 1/4 teaspoon paprika

Instructions:

1. Preheat the oven to 375°F (190°C).
2. Place the haddock fillets in a baking dish.
3. Drizzle with olive oil and sprinkle with minced garlic and paprika.
4. Top with lemon slices, olives, and capers.
5. Bake for 20-25 minutes, or until the fish flakes easily with a fork.
6. Garnish with fresh parsley before serving.

Nutrition Info (per serving):

- Calories: 280
- Protein: 34g
- Carbohydrates: 3g
- Fiber: 1g
- Sugars: 0g
- Fat: 15g
- Sodium: 520mg

Number of Servings: 4
Cooking Time: 25 minutes

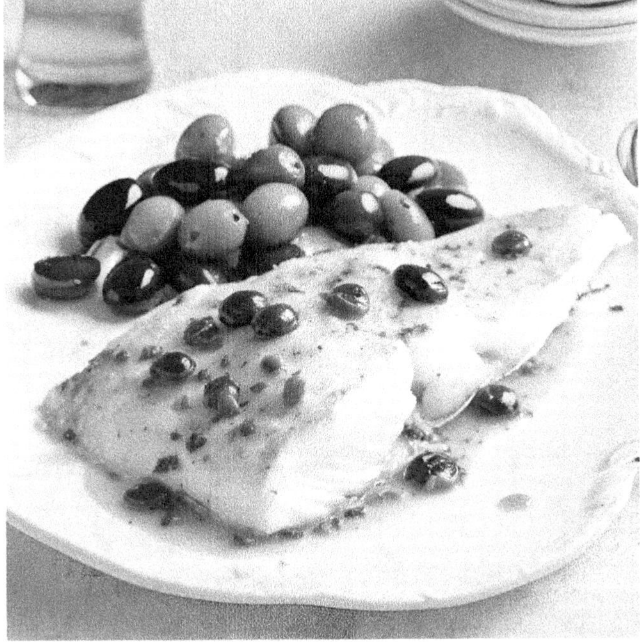

7. Steamed Clams with Basil

Ingredients:

- 2 lbs fresh clams, scrubbed clean
- 2 tablespoons olive oil
- 3 garlic cloves, minced
- 1/2 cup dry white wine
- 1/4 cup chicken broth
- 1/4 cup chopped fresh basil
- 1 tablespoon lemon juice

Instructions:

1. Heat the olive oil in a large pot over medium heat.
2. Add the garlic and cook for 1-2 minutes until fragrant.
3. Pour in the white wine and chicken broth, and bring to a simmer.
4. Add the clams, cover, and steam for 5-7 minutes, or until the clams open.
5. Discard any clams that do not open.
6. Stir in the fresh basil and lemon juice.
7. Serve immediately.

Nutrition Info (per serving):

- Calories: 200
- Protein: 22g
- Carbohydrates: 6g
- Fiber: 0g
- Sugars: 1g
- Fat: 7g
- Sodium: 540mg

Number of Servings: 4
Cooking Time: 15 minutes

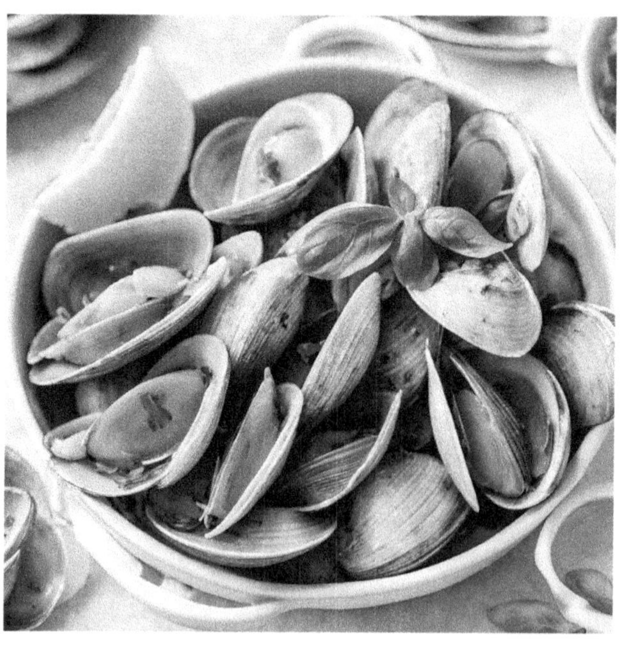

8. Fish Curry

Ingredients:

- 1 lb white fish fillets (such as cod or tilapia), cut into chunks
- 2 tablespoons olive oil
- 1 onion, chopped
- 2 garlic cloves, minced
- 1 tablespoon grated ginger
- 1 tablespoon curry powder
- 1 teaspoon ground turmeric
- 1 can (14 oz) coconut milk
- 1 cup diced tomatoes
- 1/2 cup fish broth
- 1 tablespoon lime juice
- 1/4 cup chopped fresh cilantro

Instructions:

1. Heat the olive oil in a large pot over medium heat.
2. Add the onion, garlic, and ginger, and cook for 3-5 minutes until the onion is soft.
3. Stir in the curry powder and turmeric, and cook for another 1-2 minutes.
4. Add the coconut milk, diced tomatoes, and fish broth, and bring to a simmer.
5. Add the fish chunks and cook for 5-7 minutes, or until the fish is cooked through.
6. Stir in the lime juice and garnish with fresh cilantro before serving.

Nutrition Info (per serving):

- Calories: 350
- Protein: 28g
- Carbohydrates: 10g
- Fiber: 3g
- Sugars: 4g
- Fat: 22g
- Sodium: 450mg

Number of Servings: 4
Cooking Time: 25 minutes

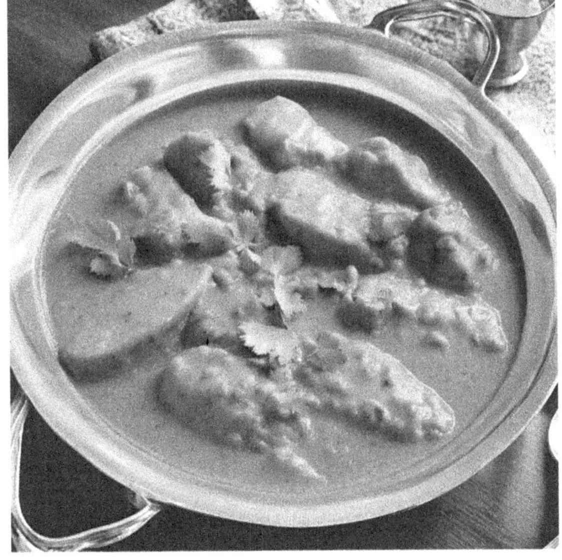

9. Shrimp Gumbo
Ingredients:

- 1 lb large shrimp, peeled and deveined
- 2 tablespoons olive oil
- 1/4 cup all-purpose flour
- 1 onion, chopped
- 1 bell pepper, chopped
- 2 celery stalks, chopped
- 2 garlic cloves, minced
- 1 can (14 oz) diced tomatoes
- 4 cups chicken broth
- 1 teaspoon dried thyme
- 1 teaspoon paprika
- 1 bay leaf
- 1/4 cup chopped fresh parsley

Instructions:

1. In a large pot, heat the olive oil over medium heat.
2. Stir in the flour to make a roux and cook, stirring constantly, until it turns a light brown color, about 5-7 minutes.
3. Add the onion, bell pepper, celery, and garlic. Cook for 5-7 minutes until the vegetables are tender.
4. Stir in the diced tomatoes, chicken broth, thyme, paprika, and bay leaf. Bring to a simmer and cook for 20 minutes.
5. Add the shrimp and cook for another 5 minutes, or until the shrimp are pink and cooked through.
6. Discard the bay leaf and garnish with fresh parsley before serving.

Nutrition Info (per serving):

- Calories: 280
- Protein: 24g
- Carbohydrates: 20g
- Fiber: 3g
- Sugars: 6g
- Fat: 12g
- Sodium: 750mg

Number of Servings: 4
Cooking Time: 35 minutes

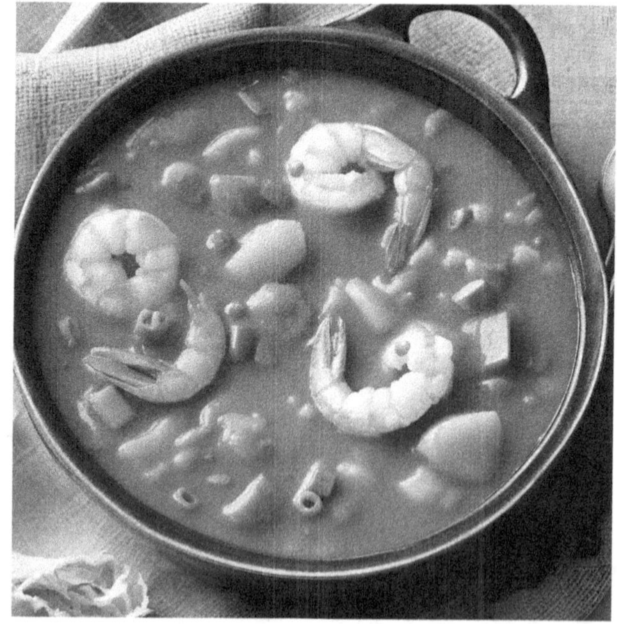

10. Paella with Seafood

Ingredients:

- 1 cup Arborio rice
- 2 tablespoons olive oil
- 1 onion, chopped
- 1 red bell pepper, chopped
- 2 garlic cloves, minced
- 1/2 teaspoon paprika
- 1/4 teaspoon saffron threads
- 1/4 teaspoon turmeric
- 1 cup diced tomatoes
- 3 cups chicken broth
- 1/2 lb large shrimp, peeled and deveined
- 1/2 lb mussels, scrubbed and debearded
- 1/2 lb squid rings
- 1/2 cup frozen peas
- 1/4 cup chopped fresh parsley
- 1 lemon, cut into wedges

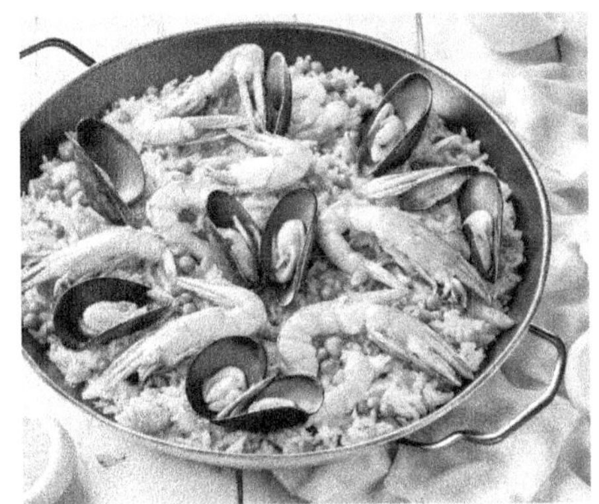

Instructions:

1. In a large, deep skillet or paella pan, heat the olive oil over medium heat.
2. Add the onion, bell pepper, and garlic, and cook for 5-7 minutes until the vegetables are tender.
3. Stir in the rice, paprika, saffron, and turmeric, and cook for 2 minutes, stirring constantly.
4. Add the diced tomatoes and chicken broth, and bring to a simmer. Cook for 15 minutes, stirring occasionally.
5. Add the shrimp, mussels, and squid. Cook for another 5-7 minutes, or until the seafood is cooked through and the mussels have opened.
6. Stir in the frozen peas and cook for another 2 minutes.
7. Garnish with chopped parsley and serve with lemon wedges.

Nutrition Info (per serving):

- Calories: 400
- Protein: 30g
- Carbohydrates: 45g
- Fiber: 4g
- Sugars: 8g
- Fat: 10g
- Sodium: 800mg

Number of Servings: 4
Cooking Time: 35 minutes

11. Sardines on Toast

Ingredients:

- 4 slices whole-grain bread
- 2 cans (4 oz each) sardines in olive oil, drained
- 1 tablespoon lemon juice
- 1 teaspoon lemon zest
- 1/4 teaspoon paprika
- 2 tablespoons chopped fresh parsley
- 1 garlic clove, minced

Instructions:

1. Toast the whole-grain bread slices.
2. In a bowl, combine the sardines, lemon juice, lemon zest, paprika, chopped parsley, and minced garlic.
3. Mash the mixture with a fork until well combined.
4. Spread the sardine mixture evenly onto the toasted bread slices.
5. Serve immediately.

Nutrition Info (per serving):

- Calories: 250
- Protein: 15g
- Carbohydrates: 20g
- Fiber: 3g
- Sugars: 1g
- Fat: 12g
- Sodium: 300mg

Number of Servings: 4

Cooking Time: 10 minutes

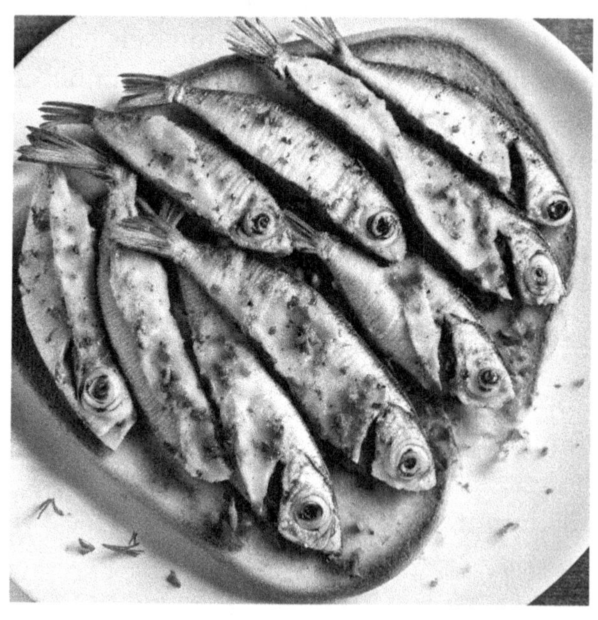

12. Oyster Stew

Ingredients:

- 1 pint shucked oysters with liquid
- 2 tablespoons unsalted butter
- 1 small onion, finely chopped
- 1 celery stalk, finely chopped
- 1 garlic clove, minced
- 2 cups whole milk
- 1 cup heavy cream
- 1/4 teaspoon paprika
- 1 tablespoon chopped fresh parsley

Instructions:

1. In a large pot, melt the butter over medium heat.
2. Add the chopped onion, celery, and garlic, and cook for 5-7 minutes until the vegetables are tender.
3. Add the oysters with their liquid, whole milk, and heavy cream.
4. Stir in the paprika and cook for 5-7 minutes, or until the oysters are cooked through and the stew is heated.
5. Garnish with chopped fresh parsley before serving.

Nutrition Info (per serving):

- Calories: 350
- Protein: 12g
- Carbohydrates: 10g
- Fiber: 1g
- Sugars: 8g
- Fat: 28g
- Sodium: 380mg

Number of Servings: 4
Cooking Time: 20 minutes

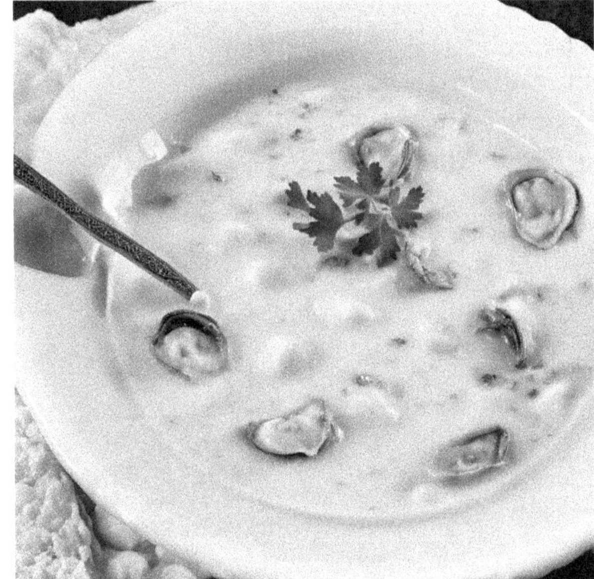

13. Squid Salad

Ingredients:

- 1 lb squid, cleaned and cut into rings
- 2 tablespoons olive oil
- 1 lemon, juiced
- 1 teaspoon lemon zest
- 2 garlic cloves, minced
- 1 cup cherry tomatoes, halved
- 1/2 cup sliced cucumber
- 1/4 cup chopped fresh parsley

Instructions:

1. Bring a large pot of water to a boil. Add the squid rings and cook for 2-3 minutes, until tender. Drain and set aside.
2. In a large bowl, whisk together the olive oil, lemon juice, lemon zest, and minced garlic.
3. Add the cooked squid, cherry tomatoes, cucumber, and chopped parsley to the bowl. Toss to coat.
4. Serve immediately.

Nutrition Info (per serving):

- Calories: 200
- Protein: 20g
- Carbohydrates: 6g
- Fiber: 1g
- Sugars: 2g
- Fat: 12g
- Sodium: 280mg

Number of Servings: 4
Cooking Time: 10 minutes

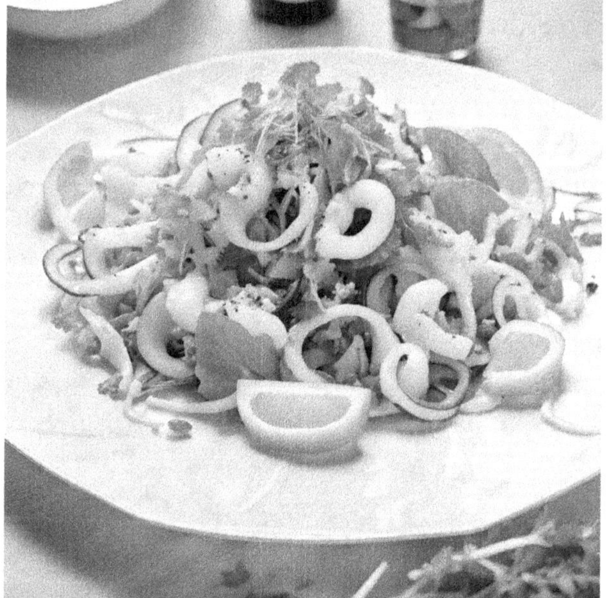

14. Fish Pie

Ingredients:

- 1 lb white fish fillets (such as cod or haddock), cut into chunks
- 1/2 cup shrimp, peeled and deveined
- 1 cup frozen peas
- 2 cups mashed potatoes
- 2 tablespoons unsalted butter
- 1 onion, chopped
- 1 carrot, diced
- 1 celery stalk, diced
- 2 tablespoons all-purpose flour
- 1 1/2 cups milk
- 1/4 teaspoon nutmeg
- 1/4 cup grated cheddar cheese

Instructions:

1. Preheat the oven to 375°F (190°C).
2. In a large skillet, melt the butter over medium heat. Add the chopped onion, carrot, and celery, and cook for 5-7 minutes until the vegetables are tender.
3. Stir in the flour and cook for 1-2 minutes.
4. Gradually add the milk, stirring constantly until the sauce thickens.
5. Stir in the nutmeg, fish chunks, shrimp, and frozen peas. Cook for 3-4 minutes until the fish and shrimp are just cooked through.
6. Pour the mixture into a baking dish and spread the mashed potatoes on top.
7. Sprinkle with grated cheddar cheese.
8. Bake for 25-30 minutes, or until the top is golden brown and the filling is bubbling.
9. Serve warm.

Nutrition Info (per serving):

- Calories: 350
- Protein: 20g
- Carbohydrates: 35g
- Fiber: 5g
- Sugars: 8g
- Fat: 15g
- Sodium: 400mg

Number of Servings: 4
Cooking Time: 45 minutes

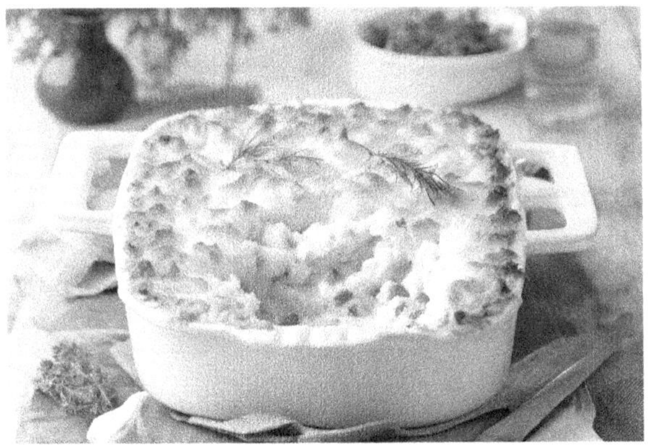

15. Crab Cakes with Remoulade Sauce

Ingredients for Crab Cakes:

- 1 lb lump crab meat
- 1/2 cup breadcrumbs
- 1 egg, beaten
- 1/4 cup mayonnaise
- 1 tablespoon Dijon mustard
- 1 tablespoon lemon juice
- 1 teaspoon Worcestershire sauce
- 2 tablespoons chopped fresh parsley
- 1/4 teaspoon paprika
- 2 tablespoons olive oil

Ingredients for Remoulade Sauce:

- 1/2 cup mayonnaise
- 1 tablespoon Dijon mustard
- 1 tablespoon lemon juice
- 1 tablespoon capers, chopped
- 1 tablespoon chopped pickles
- 1 teaspoon paprika
- 1/2 teaspoon garlic powder

Instructions:

1. In a large bowl, combine the crab meat, breadcrumbs, beaten egg, mayonnaise, Dijon mustard, lemon juice, Worcestershire sauce, chopped parsley, and paprika. Mix gently until well combined.
2. Form the mixture into 8 patties.
3. Heat the olive oil in a large skillet over medium heat. Cook the crab cakes for 3-4 minutes on each side, until golden brown and cooked through.
4. In a small bowl, mix together all the ingredients for the remoulade sauce.
5. Serve the crab cakes with the remoulade sauce on the side.

Nutrition Info (per serving):

- Calories: 300
- Protein: 20g
- Carbohydrates: 10g
- Fiber: 1g
- Sugars: 2g
- Fat: 22g
- Sodium: 450mg

Number of Servings: 4
Cooking Time: 20 minutes

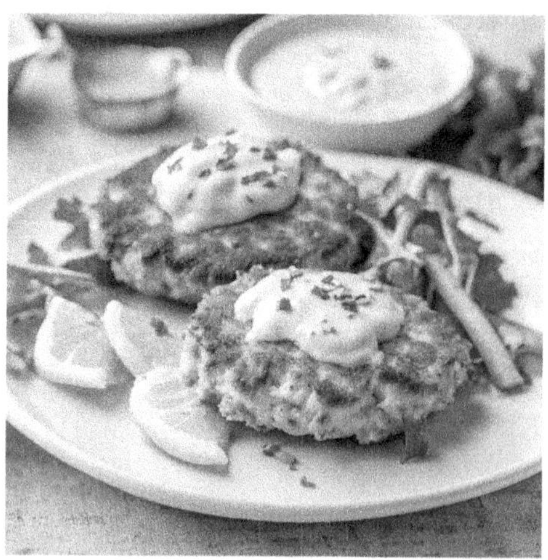

16. Lobster Tail with Herb Butter

Ingredients:

- 4 lobster tails (about 6 oz each)
- 4 tablespoons unsalted butter, melted
- 2 tablespoons lemon juice
- 2 tablespoons chopped fresh parsley
- 1 garlic clove, minced
- 1 teaspoon paprika

Instructions:

1. Preheat the oven to 425°F (220°C).
2. Using kitchen shears, cut the top of the lobster shells lengthwise, and pull the meat out slightly.
3. In a small bowl, mix the melted butter, lemon juice, chopped parsley, minced garlic, and paprika.
4. Brush the lobster meat with the herb butter mixture.
5. Place the lobster tails on a baking sheet and bake for 10-12 minutes, or until the lobster meat is opaque and cooked through.
6. Serve immediately with any remaining herb butter.

Nutrition Info (per serving):

- Calories: 280
- Protein: 24g
- Carbohydrates: 2g
- Fiber: 0g
- Sugars: 0g
- Fat: 20g
- Sodium: 300mg

Number of Servings: 4
Cooking Time: 12 minutes

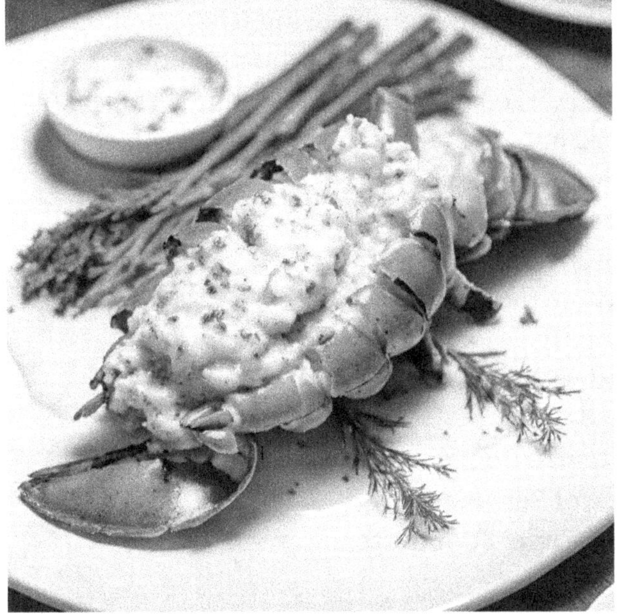

17. Spicy Tuna Roll
Ingredients:
- 1 cup sushi rice
- 1 1/4 cups water
- 2 tablespoons rice vinegar
- 1 tablespoon sugar
- 1/2 teaspoon salt
- 1/2 lb sashimi-grade tuna, diced
- 1 tablespoon Sriracha sauce
- 1 tablespoon mayonnaise
- 4 sheets nori (seaweed)
- 1/2 avocado, sliced
- 1/2 cucumber, julienned

Instructions:
1. Rinse the sushi rice under cold water until the water runs clear. Combine the rice and water in a rice cooker or saucepan and cook according to the package instructions.
2. In a small bowl, mix the rice vinegar, sugar, and salt. Fold this mixture into the cooked rice and let it cool.
3. In another bowl, combine the diced tuna, Sriracha sauce, and mayonnaise.
4. Place a sheet of nori on a bamboo sushi mat, shiny side down. Spread a thin layer of the cooled sushi rice over the nori, leaving a 1-inch border at the top.
5. Arrange a line of the tuna mixture, avocado slices, and cucumber julienne along the bottom edge of the rice.
6. Roll the sushi tightly using the bamboo mat, pressing gently to form a compact roll. Repeat with the remaining ingredients.
7. Cut each roll into 6-8 pieces using a sharp knife.
8. Serve immediately with soy sauce, pickled ginger, and wasabi if desired.

Nutrition Info (per serving):
- Calories: 250
- Protein: 18g
- Carbohydrates: 28g
- Fiber: 3g
- Sugars: 2g
- Fat: 8g
- Sodium: 200mg

Number of Servings: 4
Cooking Time: 30 minutes

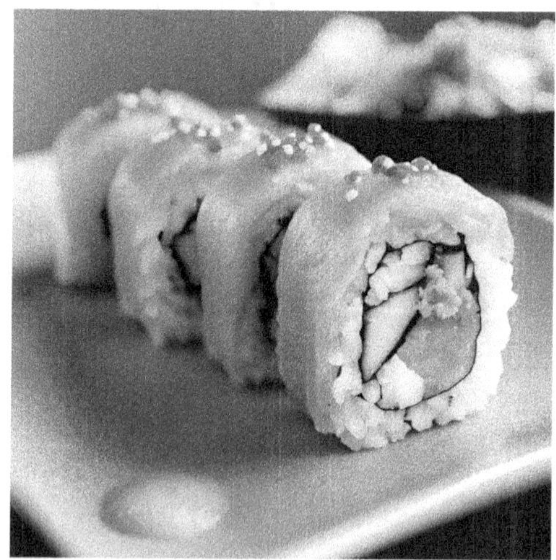

18. Poached Pear and Salmon

Ingredients:

- 4 salmon fillets (about 6 oz each)
- 2 pears, peeled, cored, and halved
- 4 cups water
- 1 cup white wine
- 1 tablespoon honey
- 1 cinnamon stick
- 2 star anise
- 1 tablespoon fresh thyme, chopped

Instructions:

1. In a large pot, combine the water, white wine, honey, cinnamon stick, and star anise. Bring to a boil, then reduce to a simmer.
2. Add the pear halves to the pot and poach for 10-15 minutes, until tender. Remove the pears and set aside.
3. Add the salmon fillets to the poaching liquid and simmer for 8-10 minutes, or until the salmon is opaque and cooked through.
4. Remove the salmon from the poaching liquid and place on a serving plate.
5. Slice the poached pears and arrange them around the salmon fillets.
6. Sprinkle with fresh thyme and serve immediately.

Nutrition Info (per serving):

- Calories: 300
- Protein: 28g
- Carbohydrates: 15g
- Fiber: 3g
- Sugars: 10g
- Fat: 12g
- Sodium: 100mg

Number of Servings: 4
Cooking Time: 25 minutes

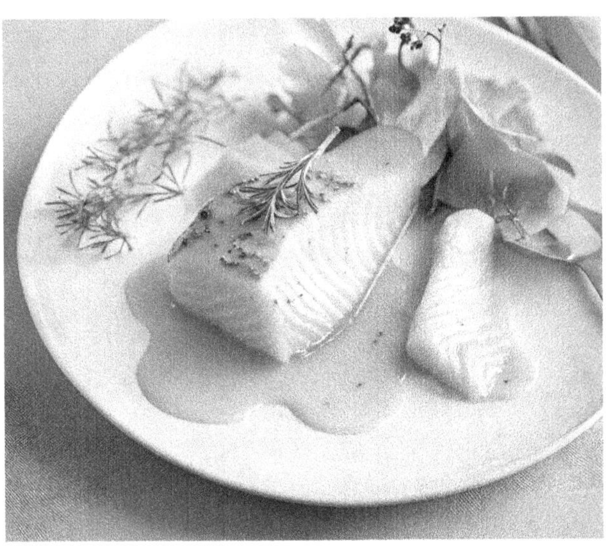

19. Ceviche

Ingredients:

- 1 lb fresh white fish (such as sea bass or tilapia), diced
- 1/2 cup lime juice
- 1/2 cup lemon juice
- 1/4 cup orange juice
- 1 red onion, finely chopped
- 1 jalapeno, seeded and finely chopped
- 1/2 cup chopped fresh cilantro
- 1 avocado, diced
- 1/2 cup cherry tomatoes, halved

Instructions:

1. In a large bowl, combine the diced fish, lime juice, lemon juice, and orange juice. Mix well and refrigerate for at least 1 hour, or until the fish is opaque and "cooked" in the citrus juices.
2. Drain off most of the marinade, leaving just a small amount.
3. Add the chopped red onion, jalapeno, cilantro, avocado, and cherry tomatoes to the fish. Mix gently to combine.
4. Serve immediately with tortilla chips or lettuce cups.

Nutrition Info (per serving):

- Calories: 200
- Protein: 20g
- Carbohydrates: 12g
- Fiber: 5g
- Sugars: 5g
- Fat: 8g
- Sodium: 150mg

Number of Servings: 4

Cooking Time: 1 hour 15 minutes

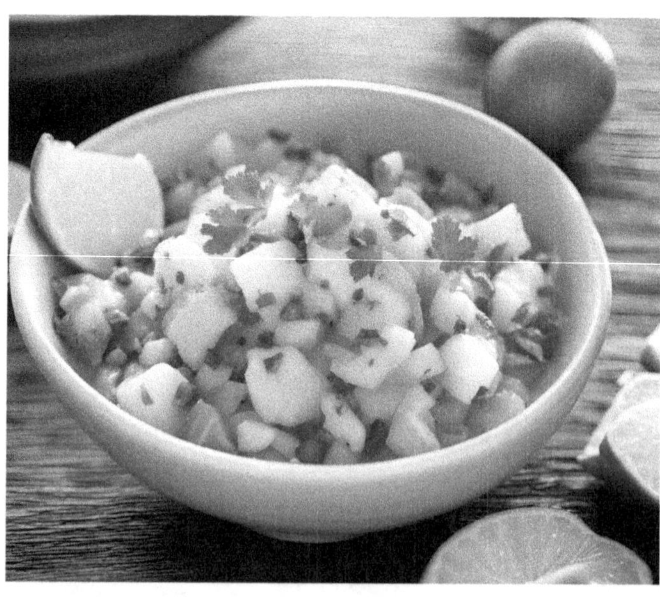

20. Ginger Soy Glazed Halibut

Ingredients:

- 4 halibut fillets (about 6 oz each)
- 2 tablespoons soy sauce
- 2 tablespoons honey
- 1 tablespoon grated fresh ginger
- 1 tablespoon rice vinegar
- 1 garlic clove, minced
- 1 tablespoon olive oil
- 2 tablespoons chopped green onions

Instructions:

1. In a small bowl, whisk together the soy sauce, honey, grated ginger, rice vinegar, and minced garlic.
2. Heat the olive oil in a large skillet over medium heat.
3. Add the halibut fillets to the skillet and cook for 3-4 minutes on each side, until golden brown and cooked through.
4. Pour the ginger soy glaze over the halibut and cook for another 1-2 minutes, until the glaze thickens.
5. Sprinkle with chopped green onions and serve immediately.

Nutrition Info (per serving):

- Calories: 280
- Protein: 34g
- Carbohydrates: 10g
- Fiber: 0g
- Sugars: 7g
- Fat: 10g
- Sodium: 450mg

Number of Servings: 4
Cooking Time: 15 minutes

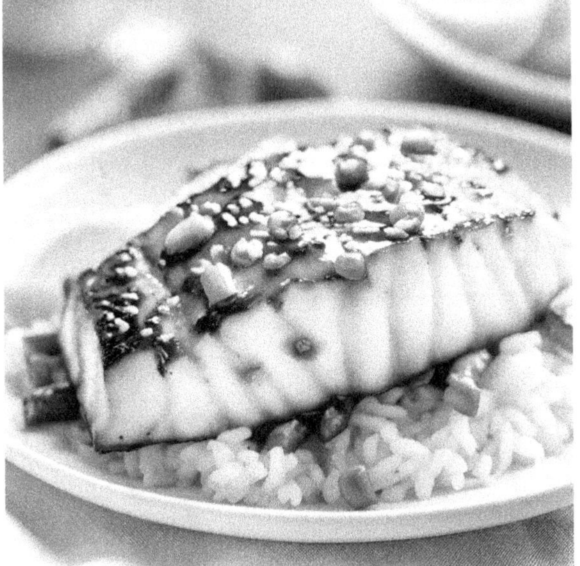

21. Pesto Shrimp Pasta

Ingredients:

- 8 oz whole wheat pasta
- 1 lb large shrimp, peeled and deveined
- 2 tablespoons olive oil
- 2 cups fresh basil leaves
- 1/4 cup pine nuts
- 1/4 cup grated Parmesan cheese
- 2 garlic cloves
- 1/2 cup olive oil
- 1/2 cup cherry tomatoes, halved

Instructions:

1. Cook the whole wheat pasta according to package instructions. Drain and set aside.
2. In a food processor, combine the basil leaves, pine nuts, Parmesan cheese, and garlic. Pulse until finely chopped.
3. With the food processor running, slowly add the olive oil until the pesto is smooth.
4. Heat 2 tablespoons of olive oil in a large skillet over medium heat. Add the shrimp and cook for 3-4 minutes, until pink and cooked through.
5. Toss the cooked pasta with the pesto, shrimp, and cherry tomatoes.
6. Serve immediately.

Nutrition Info (per serving):

- Calories: 450
- Protein: 28g
- Carbohydrates: 40g
- Fiber: 6g
- Sugars: 3g
- Fat: 20g
- Sodium: 400mg

Number of Servings: 4
Cooking Time: 20 minutes

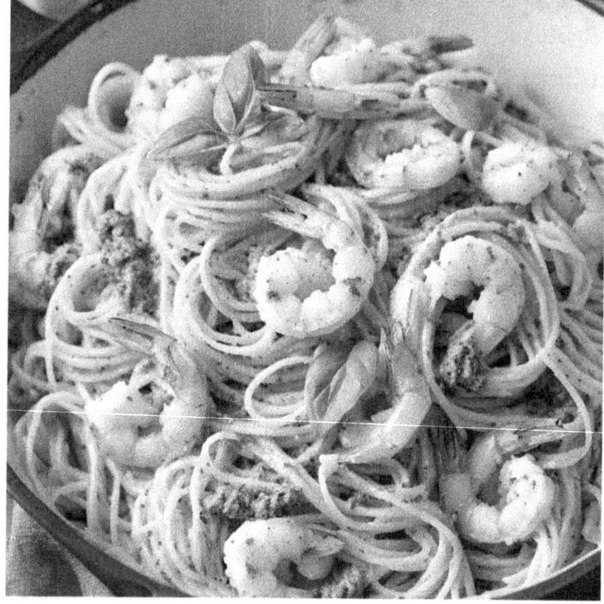

22. Shrimp and Spinach Salad

Ingredients:

- 1 lb large shrimp, peeled and deveined
- 2 tablespoons olive oil
- 1 garlic clove, minced
- 6 cups fresh spinach leaves
- 1 cup cherry tomatoes, halved
- 1/2 cucumber, sliced
- 1/4 red onion, thinly sliced
- 1 avocado, sliced
- 1/4 cup feta cheese, crumbled
- 1/4 cup balsamic vinaigrette

Instructions:

1. Heat the olive oil in a large skillet over medium heat. Add the minced garlic and cook for 1-2 minutes until fragrant.
2. Add the shrimp to the skillet and cook for 3-4 minutes, until pink and cooked through. Remove from heat and set aside.
3. In a large bowl, combine the spinach, cherry tomatoes, cucumber, red onion, avocado, and feta cheese.
4. Top with the cooked shrimp and drizzle with balsamic vinaigrette.
5. Toss gently to combine and serve immediately.

Nutrition Info (per serving):

- Calories: 300
- Protein: 25g
- Carbohydrates: 12g
- Fiber: 5g
- Sugars: 5g
- Fat: 18g
- Sodium: 450mg

Number of Servings: 4
Cooking Time: 15 minutes

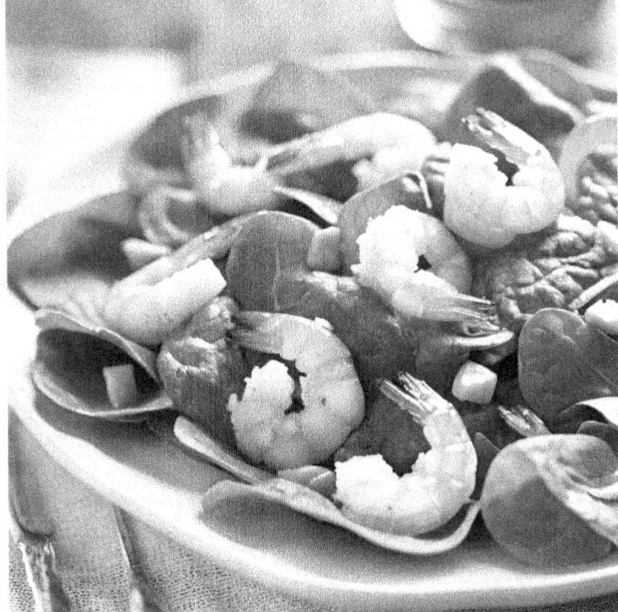

23. Baked Trout with Almonds

Ingredients:

- 4 trout fillets (about 6 oz each)
- 2 tablespoons olive oil
- 1/4 cup sliced almonds
- 1 lemon, thinly sliced
- 1 garlic clove, minced
- 2 tablespoons fresh parsley, chopped
- 1 teaspoon paprika

Instructions:

1. Preheat the oven to 375°F (190°C).
2. Place the trout fillets on a baking sheet lined with parchment paper.
3. Drizzle with olive oil and sprinkle with minced garlic and paprika.
4. Top with lemon slices and sliced almonds.
5. Bake for 15-20 minutes, or until the fish flakes easily with a fork.
6. Garnish with fresh parsley and serve immediately.

Nutrition Info (per serving):

- Calories: 300
- Protein: 34g
- Carbohydrates: 4g
- Fiber: 1g
- Sugars: 0g
- Fat: 16g
- Sodium: 90mg

Number of Servings: 4
Cooking Time: 20 minutes

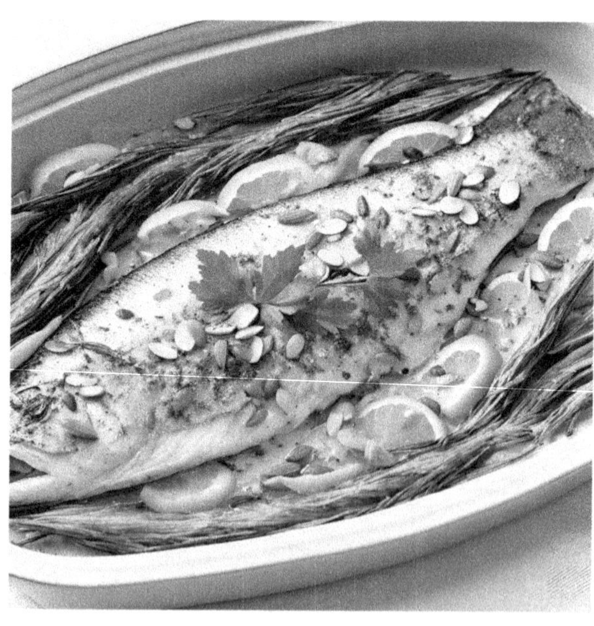

Poultry Recipes

1. Grilled Chicken Salad with Mixed Greens

Ingredients:

- 2 boneless, skinless chicken breasts
- 2 tablespoons olive oil
- 1 teaspoon dried oregano
- 1 teaspoon garlic powder
- 8 cups mixed salad greens
- 1 cup cherry tomatoes, halved
- 1/2 cucumber, sliced
- 1/4 red onion, thinly sliced
- 1/4 cup crumbled feta cheese
- 1/4 cup balsamic vinaigrette

Instructions:

1. Preheat the grill to medium-high heat.
2. In a small bowl, mix olive oil, oregano, and garlic powder.
3. Brush the chicken breasts with the olive oil mixture.
4. Grill the chicken for 6-7 minutes per side, or until cooked through. Remove from heat and let rest for 5 minutes before slicing.
5. In a large bowl, combine mixed greens, cherry tomatoes, cucumber, red onion, and feta cheese.
6. Top with grilled chicken slices and drizzle with balsamic vinaigrette.
7. Toss gently and serve immediately.

Nutrition Info (per serving):

- Calories: 300
- Protein: 28g
- Carbohydrates: 10g
- Fiber: 4g
- Sugars: 5g
- Fat: 18g
- Sodium: 320mg

Number of Servings: 4
Cooking Time: 20 minutes

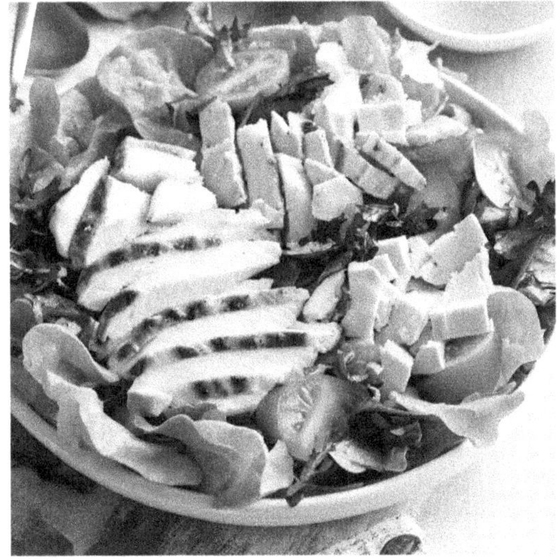

2. Turkey Meatballs in Tomato Sauce

Ingredients:

- 1 lb ground turkey
- 1/4 cup breadcrumbs
- 1 egg, beaten
- 2 tablespoons grated Parmesan cheese
- 1 teaspoon dried oregano
- 1 teaspoon garlic powder
- 2 tablespoons olive oil
- 1 onion, chopped
- 2 garlic cloves, minced
- 1 can (28 oz) crushed tomatoes
- 1 teaspoon dried basil
- 1/4 teaspoon red pepper flakes
- 2 tablespoons fresh parsley, chopped

Instructions:

1. In a large bowl, combine ground turkey, breadcrumbs, beaten egg, Parmesan cheese, oregano, and garlic powder. Mix well and form into meatballs.
2. Heat olive oil in a large skillet over medium heat. Add meatballs and cook until browned on all sides, about 5-7 minutes.
3. Remove meatballs from the skillet and set aside.
4. In the same skillet, add chopped onion and minced garlic. Cook for 3-4 minutes until softened.
5. Stir in crushed tomatoes, basil, and red pepper flakes. Bring to a simmer.
6. Return meatballs to the skillet, cover, and simmer for 20 minutes, or until meatballs are cooked through.
7. Garnish with fresh parsley and serve.

Nutrition Info (per serving):

- Calories: 280
- Protein: 28g
- Carbohydrates: 14g
- Fiber: 3g
- Sugars: 8g
- Fat: 12g
- Sodium: 400mg

Number of Servings: 4

Cooking Time: 35 minutes

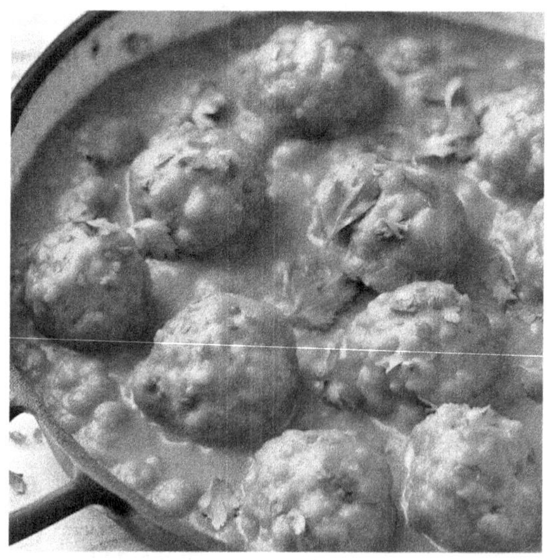

3. Baked Lemon Pepper Chicken

Ingredients:

- 4 boneless, skinless chicken breasts
- 2 tablespoons olive oil
- 1 tablespoon lemon juice
- 1 teaspoon lemon zest
- 1 teaspoon garlic powder
- 1 teaspoon dried thyme
- 1/2 teaspoon ground black pepper

Instructions:

1. Preheat the oven to 375°F (190°C).
2. In a small bowl, mix olive oil, lemon juice, lemon zest, garlic powder, dried thyme, and black pepper.
3. Place the chicken breasts in a baking dish and brush with the olive oil mixture.
4. Bake for 25-30 minutes, or until the chicken is cooked through and reaches an internal temperature of 165°F (74°C).
5. Serve immediately.

Nutrition Info (per serving):

- Calories: 250
- Protein: 34g
- Carbohydrates: 1g
- Fiber: 0g
- Sugars: 0g
- Fat: 12g
- Sodium: 100mg

Number of Servings: 4

Cooking Time: 30 minutes

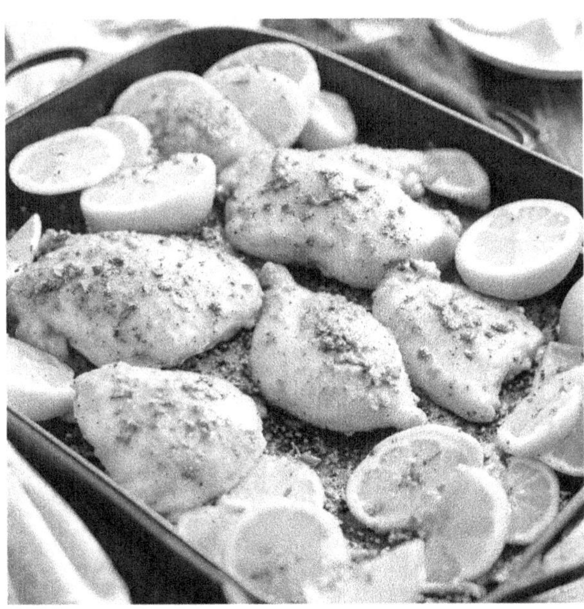

4. Chicken and Vegetable Stir-Fry

Ingredients:

- 1 lb boneless, skinless chicken breast, thinly sliced
- 2 tablespoons olive oil
- 2 garlic cloves, minced
- 1 tablespoon grated ginger
- 1 red bell pepper, sliced
- 1 yellow bell pepper, sliced
- 1 cup snap peas
- 1 cup broccoli florets
- 1/4 cup low-sodium soy sauce
- 1 tablespoon honey
- 1 tablespoon cornstarch mixed with 2 tablespoons water
- 2 tablespoons chopped fresh cilantro

Instructions:

1. Heat olive oil in a large skillet or wok over medium-high heat.
2. Add minced garlic and grated ginger, and cook for 1-2 minutes until fragrant.
3. Add the chicken slices and cook until browned and cooked through, about 5-7 minutes. Remove chicken from the skillet and set aside.
4. In the same skillet, add red bell pepper, yellow bell pepper, snap peas, and broccoli. Stir-fry for 5-6 minutes until the vegetables are tender-crisp.
5. Return the chicken to the skillet.
6. In a small bowl, mix soy sauce and honey. Pour over the chicken and vegetables, stirring to coat evenly.
7. Add the cornstarch mixture and cook for another 2-3 minutes until the sauce thickens.
8. Sprinkle with chopped fresh cilantro and serve immediately.

Nutrition Info (per serving):

- Calories: 300
- Protein: 28g
- Carbohydrates: 16g
- Fiber: 4g
- Sugars: 8g
- Fat: 14g
- Sodium: 500mg

Number of Servings: 4
Cooking Time: 20 minutes

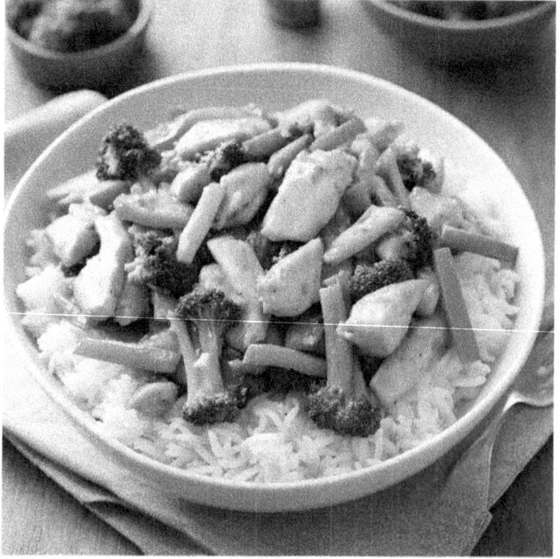

5. Turkey and Spinach Stuffed Peppers

Ingredients:

- 4 bell peppers, tops cut off and seeds removed
- 1 lb ground turkey
- 2 tablespoons olive oil
- 1 onion, chopped
- 2 garlic cloves, minced
- 4 cups fresh spinach, chopped
- 1 cup cooked quinoa
- 1 teaspoon dried oregano
- 1/2 teaspoon ground black pepper
- 1/2 cup grated Parmesan cheese

Instructions:

1. Preheat the oven to 375°F (190°C).
2. In a large skillet, heat olive oil over medium heat. Add chopped onion and minced garlic, and cook for 3-4 minutes until softened.
3. Add the ground turkey and cook until browned, about 5-7 minutes.
4. Stir in the chopped spinach, cooked quinoa, oregano, and black pepper. Cook for another 2-3 minutes until the spinach is wilted.
5. Remove from heat and stir in grated Parmesan cheese.
6. Stuff the bell peppers with the turkey and spinach mixture.
7. Place the stuffed peppers in a baking dish and cover with foil.
8. Bake for 30-35 minutes, or until the peppers are tender.
9. Serve immediately.

Nutrition Info (per serving):

- Calories: 320
- Protein: 28g
- Carbohydrates: 20g
- Fiber: 5g
- Sugars: 6g
- Fat: 14g
- Sodium: 350mg

Number of Servings: 4
Cooking Time: 40 minutes

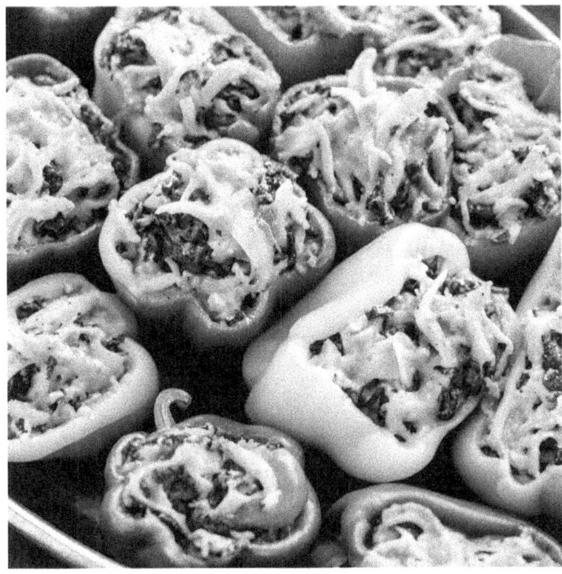

6. Chicken Noodle Soup

Ingredients:

- 1 lb boneless, skinless chicken breast, cubed
- 2 tablespoons olive oil
- 1 onion, chopped
- 3 carrots, sliced
- 2 celery stalks, sliced
- 3 garlic cloves, minced
- 8 cups low-sodium chicken broth
- 1 teaspoon dried thyme
- 1/2 teaspoon dried rosemary
- 2 cups egg noodles
- 1/4 cup chopped fresh parsley

Instructions:

1. In a large pot, heat olive oil over medium heat. Add chopped onion, carrots, celery, and minced garlic. Cook for 5-7 minutes until the vegetables are tender.
2. Add cubed chicken breast and cook until no longer pink, about 5-7 minutes.
3. Stir in the chicken broth, dried thyme, and dried rosemary. Bring to a boil.
4. Add the egg noodles and reduce heat to a simmer. Cook for 10-12 minutes until the noodles are tender.
5. Stir in chopped fresh parsley and serve immediately.

Nutrition Info (per serving):

- Calories: 250
- Protein: 25g
- Carbohydrates: 20g
- Fiber: 3g
- Sugars: 4g
- Fat: 10g
- Sodium: 350mg

Number of Servings: 6
Cooking Time: 30 minutes

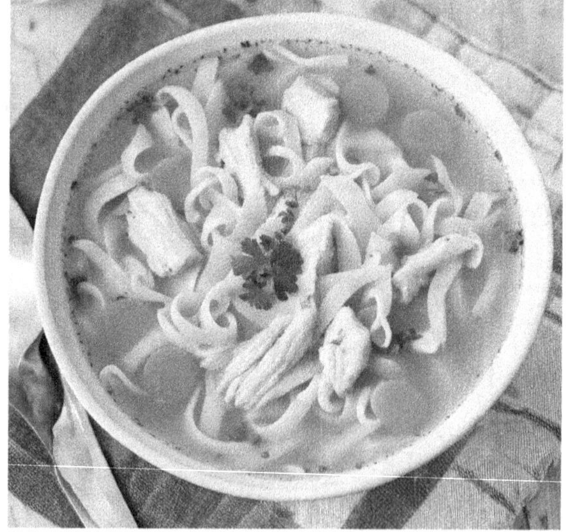

7. Chicken Caesar Wrap

Ingredients:

- 2 boneless, skinless chicken breasts
- 2 tablespoons olive oil
- 1 teaspoon garlic powder
- 1/2 teaspoon ground black pepper
- 4 whole-grain tortillas
- 4 cups chopped romaine lettuce
- 1/4 cup grated Parmesan cheese
- 1/4 cup Caesar dressing

Instructions:

1. Preheat the grill to medium-high heat.
2. In a small bowl, mix olive oil, garlic powder, and black pepper.
3. Brush the chicken breasts with the olive oil mixture.
4. Grill the chicken for 6-7 minutes per side, or until cooked through. Remove from heat and let rest for 5 minutes before slicing.
5. In a large bowl, combine chopped romaine lettuce, grated Parmesan cheese, and Caesar dressing. Toss to coat.
6. Lay out the tortillas and divide the salad mixture evenly among them.
7. Top with sliced grilled chicken.
8. Roll up the tortillas and serve immediately.

Nutrition Info (per serving):

- Calories: 350
- Protein: 28g
- Carbohydrates: 25g
- Fiber: 4g
- Sugars: 2g
- Fat: 16g
- Sodium: 500mg

Number of Servings: 4
Cooking Time: 20 minutes

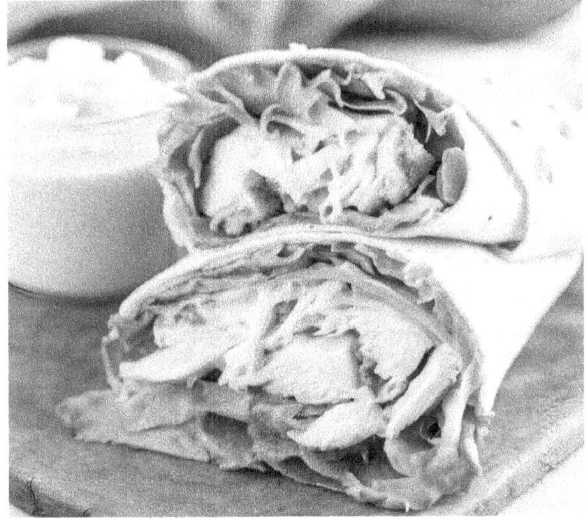

8. Smoked Turkey Breast on Rye

Ingredients:

- 8 slices rye bread
- 1 lb thinly sliced smoked turkey breast
- 4 slices Swiss cheese
- 1/4 cup Dijon mustard
- 1/4 cup mayonnaise
- 1/2 cup arugula leaves
- 1 tomato, thinly sliced

Instructions:

1. In a small bowl, mix the Dijon mustard and mayonnaise.
2. Spread the mustard mixture on each slice of rye bread.
3. Layer the smoked turkey breast, Swiss cheese, arugula leaves, and tomato slices on four of the bread slices.
4. Top with the remaining bread slices to make sandwiches.
5. Serve immediately.

Nutrition Info (per serving):

- Calories: 350
- Protein: 28g
- Carbohydrates: 30g
- Fiber: 5g
- Sugars: 3g
- Fat: 14g
- Sodium: 750mg

Number of Servings: 4

Cooking Time: 10 minutes

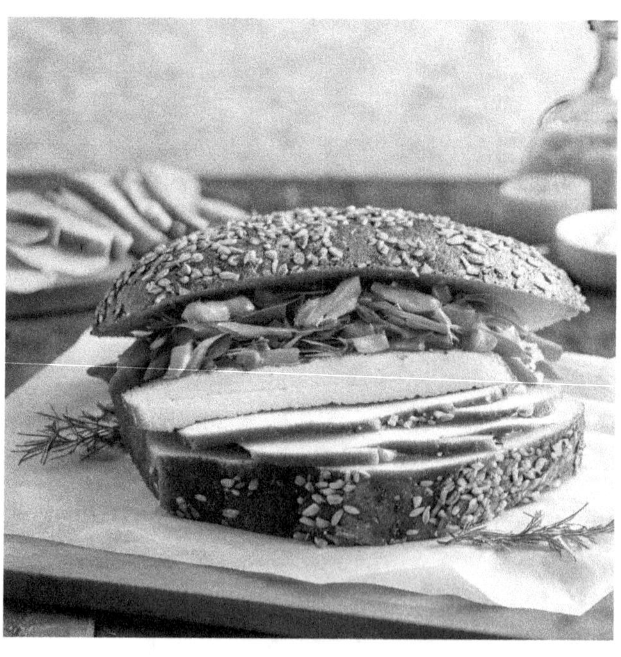

9. Grilled Chicken and Pineapple Skewers

Ingredients:

- 2 boneless, skinless chicken breasts, cut into cubes
- 1 cup pineapple chunks
- 2 tablespoons olive oil
- 1 tablespoon honey
- 1 tablespoon soy sauce
- 1 garlic clove, minced
- 1/4 teaspoon ground black pepper

Instructions:

1. In a small bowl, mix olive oil, honey, soy sauce, minced garlic, and black pepper.
2. Thread the chicken cubes and pineapple chunks onto skewers, alternating them.
3. Brush the skewers with the olive oil mixture.
4. Preheat the grill to medium-high heat.
5. Grill the skewers for 10-12 minutes, turning occasionally, until the chicken is cooked through and the pineapple is caramelized.
6. Serve immediately.

Nutrition Info (per serving):

- Calories: 250
- Protein: 28g
- Carbohydrates: 15g
- Fiber: 1g
- Sugars: 10g
- Fat: 10g
- Sodium: 200mg

Number of Servings: 4
Cooking Time: 20 minutes

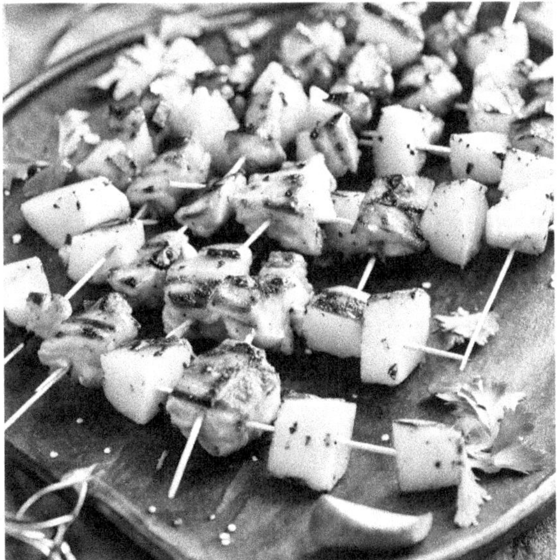

10. Slow Cooker Chicken and Lentils

Ingredients:

- 1 lb boneless, skinless chicken thighs
- 1 cup dried lentils, rinsed
- 1 onion, chopped
- 2 carrots, sliced
- 2 celery stalks, sliced
- 3 garlic cloves, minced
- 4 cups low-sodium chicken broth
- 1 teaspoon dried thyme
- 1/2 teaspoon ground black pepper
- 2 tablespoons fresh parsley, chopped

Instructions:

1. In a slow cooker, combine chicken thighs, lentils, chopped onion, carrots, celery, minced garlic, chicken broth, dried thyme, and black pepper.
2. Cover and cook on low for 6-7 hours, or until the chicken and lentils are tender.
3. Remove the chicken thighs, shred them with two forks, and return to the slow cooker.
4. Stir in the chopped fresh parsley and serve.

Nutrition Info (per serving):

- Calories: 300
- Protein: 30g
- Carbohydrates: 25g
- Fiber: 8g
- Sugars: 5g
- Fat: 10g
- Sodium: 350mg

Number of Servings: 6
Cooking Time: 7 hours

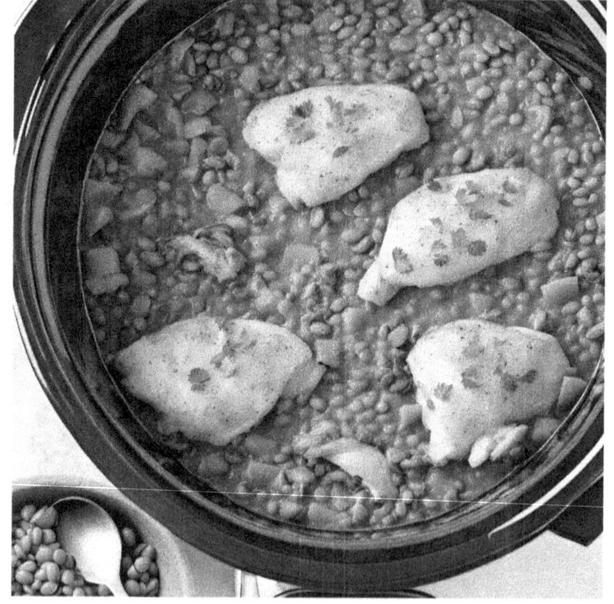

11. Chicken Vegetable Pot Pie

Ingredients:

- 1 lb boneless, skinless chicken breast, cubed
- 2 tablespoons olive oil
- 1 onion, chopped
- 2 carrots, sliced
- 2 celery stalks, sliced
- 1 cup frozen peas
- 1 cup frozen corn
- 2 garlic cloves, minced
- 2 cups low-sodium chicken broth
- 1/2 cup milk
- 1/4 cup all-purpose flour
- 1 teaspoon dried thyme
- 1/2 teaspoon ground black pepper
- 1 sheet puff pastry, thawed

Instructions:

1. Preheat the oven to 400°F (200°C).
2. In a large skillet, heat olive oil over medium heat. Add chopped onion, carrots, celery, and minced garlic. Cook for 5-7 minutes until the vegetables are tender.
3. Add the cubed chicken breast and cook until no longer pink, about 5-7 minutes.
4. Stir in the chicken broth, milk, dried thyme, and black pepper.
5. Sprinkle the flour over the mixture and stir until the sauce thickens.
6. Add the frozen peas and corn, and cook for another 2-3 minutes.
7. Pour the mixture into a baking dish and cover with the puff pastry sheet, trimming any excess.
8. Bake for 20-25 minutes, or until the pastry is golden brown.
9. Serve immediately.

Nutrition Info (per serving):

- Calories: 400
- Protein: 28g
- Carbohydrates: 35g
- Fiber: 5g
- Sugars: 6g
- Fat: 16g
- Sodium: 450mg

Number of Servings: 6

Cooking Time: 35 minutes

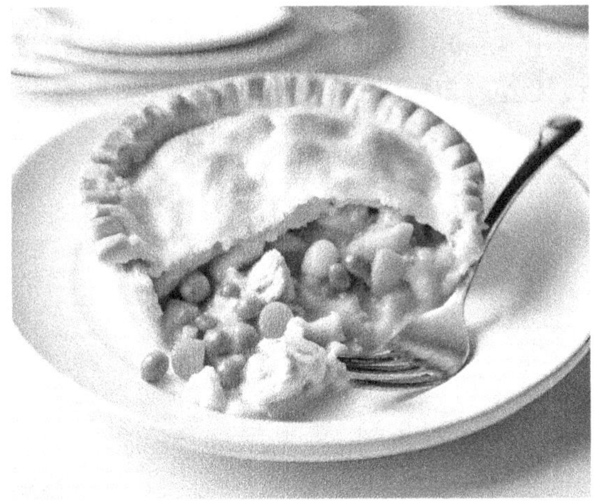

12. Chicken Fajitas

Ingredients:

- 1 lb boneless, skinless chicken breast, thinly sliced
- 2 tablespoons olive oil
- 1 onion, sliced
- 1 red bell pepper, sliced
- 1 yellow bell pepper, sliced
- 1 green bell pepper, sliced
- 2 garlic cloves, minced
- 1 teaspoon ground cumin
- 1 teaspoon chili powder
- 1/2 teaspoon ground black pepper
- 8 whole-grain tortillas
- 1/4 cup fresh cilantro, chopped
- 1 lime, cut into wedges

Instructions:

1. Heat olive oil in a large skillet over medium-high heat.
2. Add sliced onion, red bell pepper, yellow bell pepper, green bell pepper, and minced garlic. Cook for 5-7 minutes until the vegetables are tender-crisp.
3. Add the thinly sliced chicken breast, ground cumin, chili powder, and black pepper. Cook until the chicken is cooked through, about 5-7 minutes.
4. Warm the whole-grain tortillas in a dry skillet or microwave.
5. Divide the chicken and vegetable mixture among the tortillas.
6. Sprinkle with chopped fresh cilantro and serve with lime wedges.

Nutrition Info (per serving):

- Calories: 350
- Protein: 28g
- Carbohydrates: 35g
- Fiber: 6g
- Sugars: 5g
- Fat: 12g
- Sodium: 400mg

Number of Servings: 4
Cooking Time: 20 minutes

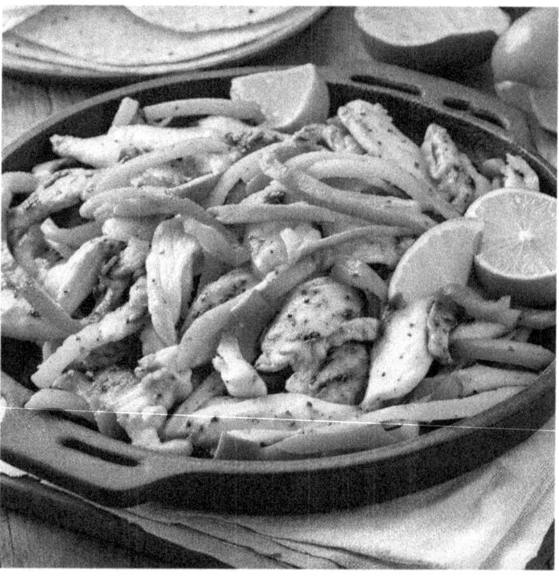

13. Asian Turkey Lettuce Wraps

Ingredients:

- 1 lb ground turkey
- 2 tablespoons olive oil
- 1 onion, finely chopped
- 2 garlic cloves, minced
- 1 tablespoon grated ginger
- 1/4 cup hoisin sauce
- 2 tablespoons soy sauce
- 1 tablespoon rice vinegar
- 1 teaspoon sesame oil
- 8 large lettuce leaves
- 1/4 cup shredded carrots
- 2 tablespoons chopped fresh cilantro

Instructions:

1. Heat olive oil in a large skillet over medium heat. Add finely chopped onion, minced garlic, and grated ginger. Cook for 3-4 minutes until the onion is soft.
2. Add the ground turkey and cook until browned, about 5-7 minutes.
3. Stir in hoisin sauce, soy sauce, rice vinegar, and sesame oil. Cook for another 2-3 minutes until the turkey is well coated and heated through.
4. Spoon the turkey mixture into the center of the lettuce leaves.
5. Top with shredded carrots and chopped fresh cilantro.
6. Serve immediately.

Nutrition Info (per serving):

- Calories: 250
- Protein: 25g
- Carbohydrates: 10g
- Fiber: 3g
- Sugars: 5g
- Fat: 12g
- Sodium: 450mg

Number of Servings: 4
Cooking Time: 15 minutes

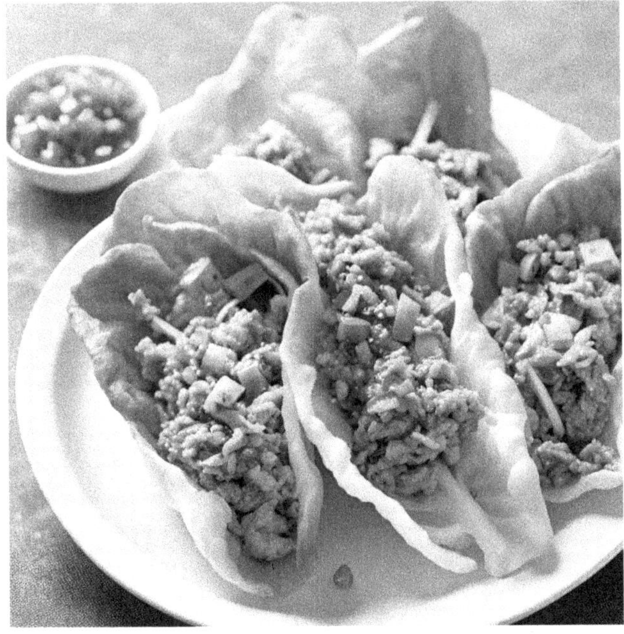

14. Paprika Chicken with Chickpeas

Ingredients:

- 4 boneless, skinless chicken breasts
- 2 tablespoons olive oil
- 1 tablespoon smoked paprika
- 1 teaspoon garlic powder
- 1 can (15 oz) chickpeas, drained and rinsed
- 1 cup cherry tomatoes, halved
- 1/4 cup chopped fresh parsley
- 1 lemon, cut into wedges

Instructions:

1. Preheat the oven to 400°F (200°C).
2. In a small bowl, mix the olive oil, smoked paprika, and garlic powder.
3. Rub the mixture over the chicken breasts and place them in a baking dish.
4. Add the chickpeas and cherry tomatoes around the chicken.
5. Bake for 25-30 minutes, or until the chicken is cooked through and reaches an internal temperature of 165°F (74°C).
6. Garnish with chopped fresh parsley and serve with lemon wedges.

Nutrition Info (per serving):

- Calories: 350
- Protein: 36g
- Carbohydrates: 20g
- Fiber: 6g
- Sugars: 2g
- Fat: 14g
- Sodium: 400mg

Number of Servings: 4
Cooking Time: 30 minutes

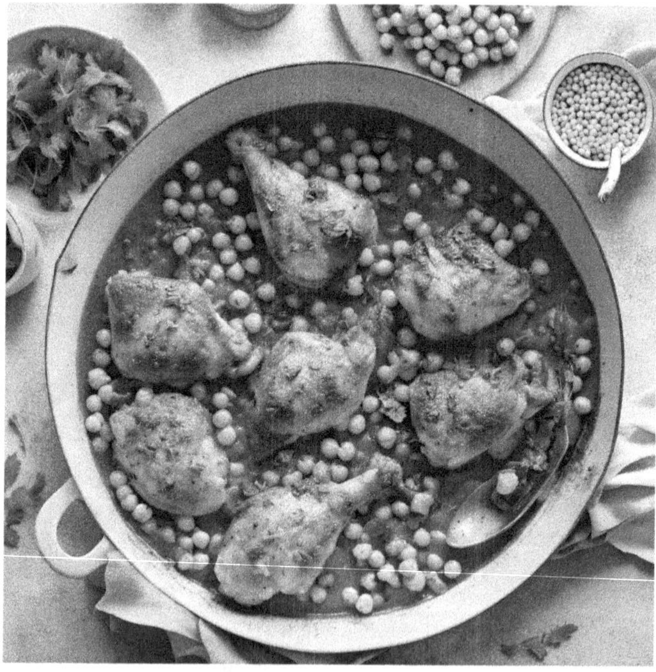

15. Roast Chicken with Root Vegetables

Ingredients:

- 1 whole chicken (4-5 lbs)
- 3 tablespoons olive oil
- 1 tablespoon dried rosemary
- 1 tablespoon dried thyme
- 4 carrots, peeled and cut into chunks
- 3 parsnips, peeled and cut into chunks
- 2 potatoes, cut into chunks
- 1 onion, quartered
- 1 lemon, halved
- 1/4 cup fresh parsley, chopped

Instructions:

1. Preheat the oven to 375°F (190°C).
2. In a small bowl, mix 2 tablespoons of olive oil with dried rosemary and thyme.
3. Rub the mixture all over the chicken.
4. Place the chicken in a roasting pan and surround it with carrots, parsnips, potatoes, and onion.
5. Drizzle the remaining olive oil over the vegetables.
6. Squeeze the lemon halves over the chicken and place the lemon halves inside the cavity.
7. Roast for 1 hour and 30 minutes, or until the chicken reaches an internal temperature of 165°F (74°C).
8. Let the chicken rest for 10 minutes before carving.
9. Garnish with chopped fresh parsley and serve.

Nutrition Info (per serving):

- Calories: 500
- Protein: 40g
- Carbohydrates: 30g
- Fiber: 6g
- Sugars: 5g
- Fat: 24g
- Sodium: 300mg

Number of Servings: 6

Cooking Time: 1 hour 40 minutes

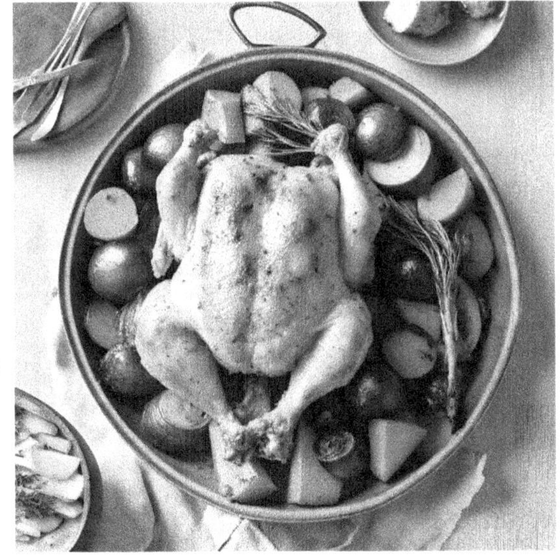

16. Chicken Tabbouleh Salad

Ingredients:

- 2 boneless, skinless chicken breasts
- 2 tablespoons olive oil
- 1 cup bulgur wheat
- 2 cups water
- 1 cup chopped fresh parsley
- 1/2 cup chopped fresh mint
- 1 cup cherry tomatoes, halved
- 1/2 cucumber, diced
- 1/4 red onion, finely chopped
- 1/4 cup lemon juice
- 2 tablespoons olive oil

Instructions:

1. Preheat the grill to medium-high heat.
2. Brush the chicken breasts with 1 tablespoon of olive oil.
3. Grill the chicken for 6-7 minutes per side, or until cooked through. Remove from heat and let rest for 5 minutes before slicing.
4. In a medium saucepan, bring the water to a boil. Stir in the bulgur wheat, cover, and remove from heat. Let sit for 15 minutes, or until the bulgur is tender and the water is absorbed. Fluff with a fork.
5. In a large bowl, combine the cooked bulgur, chopped parsley, chopped mint, cherry tomatoes, cucumber, and red onion.
6. In a small bowl, whisk together the lemon juice and 2 tablespoons of olive oil.
7. Pour the dressing over the tabbouleh and toss to combine.
8. Top with sliced grilled chicken and serve immediately.

Nutrition Info (per serving):

- Calories: 350
- Protein: 28g
- Carbohydrates: 30g
- Fiber: 6g
- Sugars: 4g
- Fat: 14g
- Sodium: 200mg

Number of Servings: 4
Cooking Time: 25 minutes

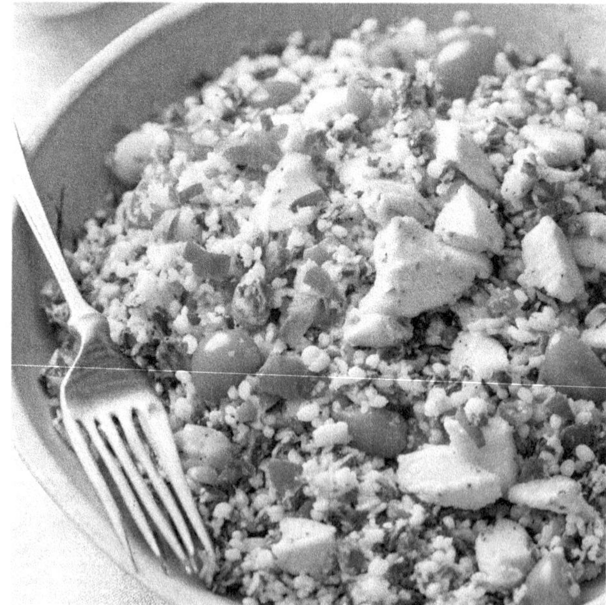

17. Balsamic Glazed Chicken Breasts

Ingredients:

- 4 boneless, skinless chicken breasts
- 2 tablespoons olive oil
- 1/4 cup balsamic vinegar
- 1/4 cup chicken broth
- 2 tablespoons honey
- 2 garlic cloves, minced
- 1 teaspoon dried thyme

Instructions:

1. Preheat the oven to 375°F (190°C).
2. Heat olive oil in a large oven-safe skillet over medium-high heat.
3. Add the chicken breasts and cook for 3-4 minutes per side, until golden brown.
4. In a small bowl, whisk together balsamic vinegar, chicken broth, honey, minced garlic, and dried thyme.
5. Pour the balsamic mixture over the chicken in the skillet.
6. Transfer the skillet to the oven and bake for 15-20 minutes, or until the chicken is cooked through and reaches an internal temperature of 165°F (74°C).
7. Remove from the oven and let rest for 5 minutes before serving.

Nutrition Info (per serving):

- Calories: 280
- Protein: 28g
- Carbohydrates: 12g
- Fiber: 0g
- Sugars: 10g
- Fat: 12g
- Sodium: 200mg

Number of Servings: 4
Cooking Time: 25 minutes

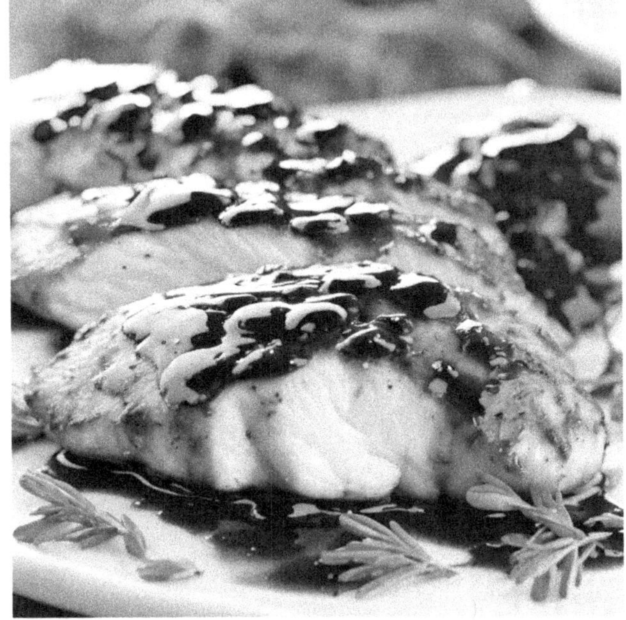

18. Greek Chicken Skewers

Ingredients:

- 2 boneless, skinless chicken breasts, cut into cubes
- 2 tablespoons olive oil
- 1 tablespoon lemon juice
- 1 teaspoon dried oregano
- 1 teaspoon garlic powder
- 1/2 teaspoon ground black pepper
- 1 red bell pepper, cut into chunks
- 1 green bell pepper, cut into chunks
- 1 red onion, cut into chunks
- 1/2 cup tzatziki sauce (for serving)

Instructions:

1. In a small bowl, mix olive oil, lemon juice, dried oregano, garlic powder, and black pepper.
2. Thread the chicken cubes, red bell pepper chunks, green bell pepper chunks, and red onion chunks onto skewers, alternating them.
3. Brush the skewers with the olive oil mixture.
4. Preheat the grill to medium-high heat.
5. Grill the skewers for 10-12 minutes, turning occasionally, until the chicken is cooked through.
6. Serve immediately with tzatziki sauce.

Nutrition Info (per serving):

- Calories: 300
- Protein: 28g
- Carbohydrates: 10g
- Fiber: 3g
- Sugars: 4g
- Fat: 16g
- Sodium: 250mg

Number of Servings: 4
Cooking Time: 20 minutes

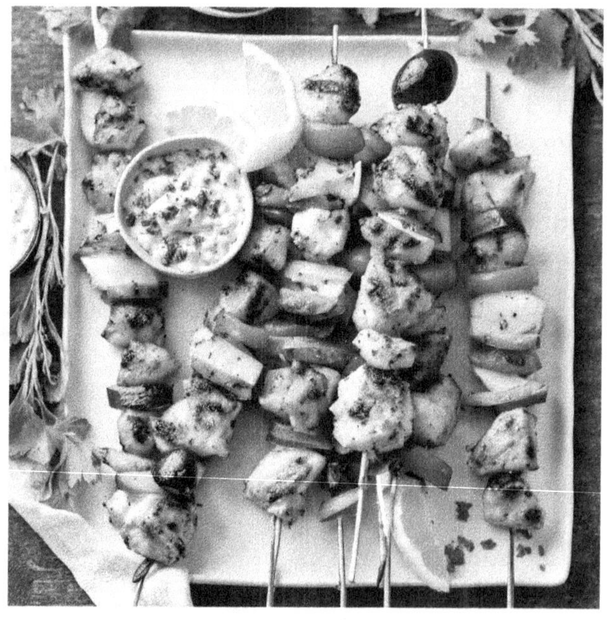

19. Chicken and Barley Soup

Ingredients:

- 1 lb boneless, skinless chicken breast, cubed
- 2 tablespoons olive oil
- 1 onion, chopped
- 3 carrots, sliced
- 2 celery stalks, sliced
- 3 garlic cloves, minced
- 8 cups low-sodium chicken broth
- 1 cup pearl barley
- 1 teaspoon dried thyme
- 1/2 teaspoon ground black pepper
- 1/4 cup chopped fresh parsley

Instructions:

1. In a large pot, heat olive oil over medium heat. Add chopped onion, carrots, celery, and minced garlic. Cook for 5-7 minutes until the vegetables are tender.
2. Add the cubed chicken breast and cook until no longer pink, about 5-7 minutes.
3. Stir in the chicken broth, pearl barley, dried thyme, and black pepper. Bring to a boil.
4. Reduce heat and simmer for 45-50 minutes, or until the barley is tender.
5. Stir in chopped fresh parsley and serve.

Nutrition Info (per serving):

- Calories: 300
- Protein: 28g
- Carbohydrates: 30g
- Fiber: 6g
- Sugars: 5g
- Fat: 8g
- Sodium: 350mg

Number of Servings: 6
Cooking Time: 1 hour

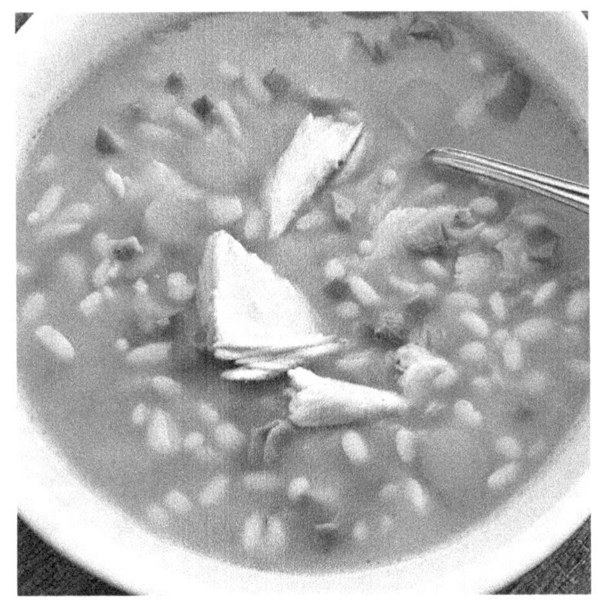

20. Turkey and Quinoa Stuffed Tomatoes

Ingredients:

- 6 large tomatoes, tops cut off and seeds removed
- 1 lb ground turkey
- 1 cup cooked quinoa
- 2 tablespoons olive oil
- 1 onion, chopped
- 2 garlic cloves, minced
- 1 teaspoon dried basil
- 1/2 teaspoon ground black pepper
- 1/4 cup grated Parmesan cheese
- 2 tablespoons chopped fresh parsley

Instructions:

1. Preheat the oven to 375°F (190°C).
2. In a large skillet, heat olive oil over medium heat. Add chopped onion and minced garlic, and cook for 3-4 minutes until softened.
3. Add the ground turkey and cook until browned, about 5-7 minutes.
4. Stir in the cooked quinoa, dried basil, and black pepper. Cook for another 2-3 minutes.
5. Remove from heat and stir in grated Parmesan cheese and chopped fresh parsley.
6. Stuff the tomatoes with the turkey and quinoa mixture.
7. Place the stuffed tomatoes in a baking dish and bake for 25-30 minutes, or until the tomatoes are tender.
8. Serve immediately.

Nutrition Info (per serving):

- Calories: 250
- Protein: 20g
- Carbohydrates: 18g
- Fiber: 4g
- Sugars: 7g
- Fat: 12g
- Sodium: 250mg

Number of Servings: 6
Cooking Time: 30 minutes

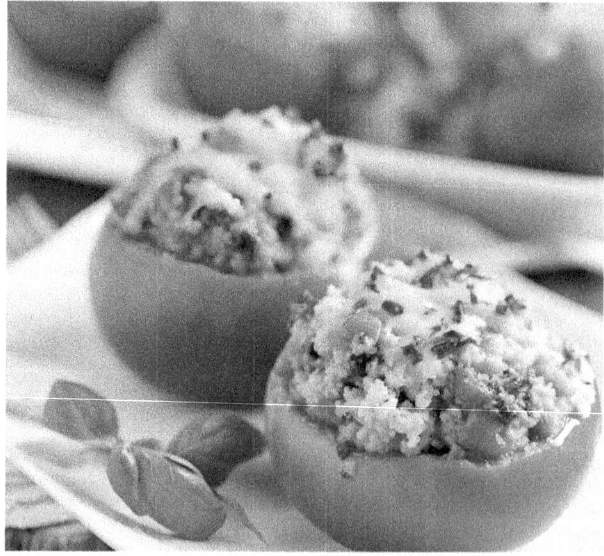

21. Chicken Piccata

Ingredients:

- 4 boneless, skinless chicken breasts
- 1/4 cup all-purpose flour
- 2 tablespoons olive oil
- 1/4 cup chicken broth
- 1/4 cup lemon juice
- 2 tablespoons capers, rinsed
- 2 tablespoons unsalted butter
- 1/4 cup chopped fresh parsley

Instructions:

1. Pound the chicken breasts to an even thickness and coat them lightly with flour.
2. Heat olive oil in a large skillet over medium-high heat. Add the chicken breasts and cook for 4-5 minutes per side, until golden brown and cooked through. Remove from heat and set aside.
3. In the same skillet, add chicken broth, lemon juice, and capers. Bring to a simmer and cook for 2-3 minutes.
4. Stir in unsalted butter until melted and smooth.
5. Return the chicken to the skillet and spoon the sauce over the top.
6. Garnish with chopped fresh parsley and serve immediately.

Nutrition Info (per serving):

- Calories: 320
- Protein: 28g
- Carbohydrates: 10g
- Fiber: 1g
- Sugars: 1g
- Fat: 18g
- Sodium: 300mg

Number of Servings: 4
Cooking Time: 20 minutes

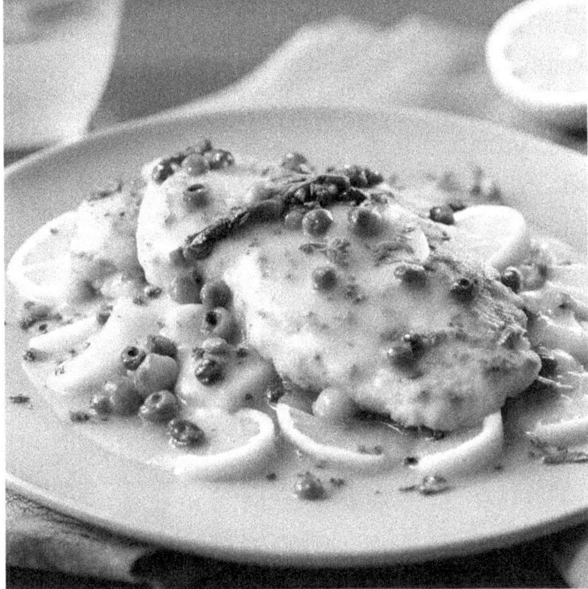

22. Chicken and Spinach Quiche

Ingredients:

- 1 pre-made pie crust
- 1 lb boneless, skinless chicken breast, cooked and diced
- 2 cups fresh spinach, chopped
- 1 cup shredded mozzarella cheese
- 1/2 cup grated Parmesan cheese
- 1 cup milk
- 4 large eggs
- 1 teaspoon dried basil
- 1/2 teaspoon ground black pepper

Instructions:

1. Preheat the oven to 375°F (190°C).
2. Place the pie crust in a pie dish and bake for 10 minutes. Remove from the oven and set aside.
3. In a large bowl, combine cooked and diced chicken breast, chopped spinach, shredded mozzarella cheese, and grated Parmesan cheese. Mix well.
4. In another bowl, whisk together milk, eggs, dried basil, and black pepper.
5. Pour the chicken and spinach mixture into the pre-baked pie crust.
6. Pour the egg mixture over the top.
7. Bake for 35-40 minutes, or until the quiche is set and the top is golden brown.
8. Let cool for 10 minutes before slicing and serving.

Nutrition Info (per serving):

- Calories: 350
- Protein: 28g
- Carbohydrates: 18g
- Fiber: 2g
- Sugars: 4g
- Fat: 20g
- Sodium: 350mg

Number of Servings: 6
Cooking Time: 50 minutes

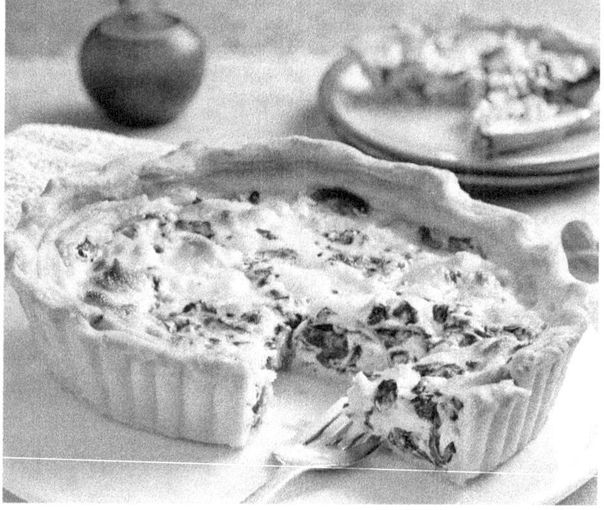

23. Moroccan Chicken with Couscous

Ingredients:

- 4 boneless, skinless chicken thighs
- 2 tablespoons olive oil
- 1 onion, chopped
- 2 garlic cloves, minced
- 1 teaspoon ground cumin
- 1 teaspoon ground cinnamon
- 1 teaspoon ground ginger
- 1/2 teaspoon ground turmeric
- 1 can (14 oz) diced tomatoes
- 1/2 cup chicken broth
- 1 cup dried apricots, chopped
- 1 cup couscous
- 1/4 cup chopped fresh cilantro

Instructions:

1. Heat olive oil in a large skillet over medium heat. Add chopped onion and minced garlic, and cook for 3-4 minutes until softened.
2. Add the chicken thighs and cook until browned, about 5-7 minutes per side. Remove from heat and set aside.
3. In the same skillet, stir in ground cumin, ground cinnamon, ground ginger, and ground turmeric. Cook for 1-2 minutes until fragrant.
4. Add diced tomatoes, chicken broth, and chopped dried apricots. Bring to a simmer.
5. Return the chicken thighs to the skillet, cover, and cook for 20-25 minutes, or until the chicken is cooked through.
6. Meanwhile, cook the couscous according to the package instructions.
7. Serve the chicken and sauce over the couscous, and garnish with chopped fresh cilantro.

Nutrition Info (per serving):

- Calories: 400
- Protein: 28g
- Carbohydrates: 45g
- Fiber: 6g
- Sugars: 15g
- Fat: 14g
- Sodium: 400mg

Number of Servings: 4
Cooking Time: 30 minutes

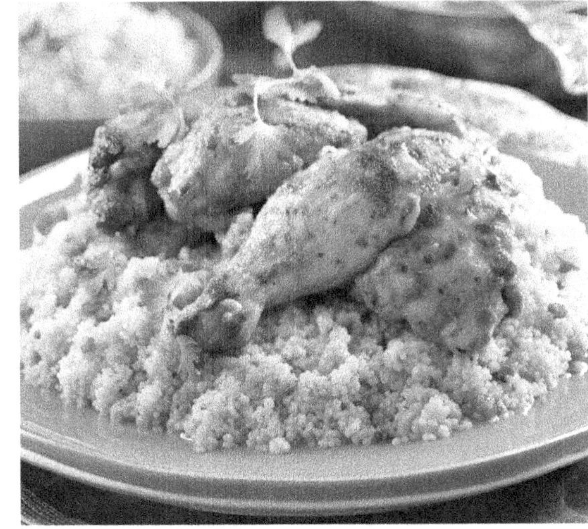

Beef and Pork Recipes

1. Slow-Cooked Beef Stew

Ingredients:

- 2 lbs beef chuck, cut into 1-inch cubes
- 2 tablespoons olive oil
- 1 onion, chopped
- 3 carrots, sliced
- 2 celery stalks, sliced
- 3 garlic cloves, minced
- 4 cups low-sodium beef broth
- 1 cup red wine (optional)
- 2 tablespoons tomato paste
- 1 teaspoon dried thyme
- 1 teaspoon dried rosemary
- 2 potatoes, peeled and diced
- 1 cup peas (frozen or fresh)

Instructions:

1. Heat the olive oil in a large skillet over medium heat. Add the beef cubes and brown on all sides, about 5-7 minutes.
2. Transfer the browned beef to a slow cooker.
3. In the same skillet, add the onion, carrots, celery, and garlic. Cook for 3-4 minutes until softened.
4. Transfer the vegetables to the slow cooker.
5. Add the beef broth, red wine (if using), tomato paste, thyme, and rosemary to the slow cooker. Stir to combine.
6. Add the diced potatoes to the slow cooker.
7. Cover and cook on low for 7-8 hours, or until the beef is tender.
8. Stir in the peas and cook for another 15-20 minutes until heated through.
9. Serve hot.

Nutrition Info (per serving):

- Calories: 350
- Protein: 28g
- Carbohydrates: 20g
- Fiber: 4g
- Sugars: 6g
- Fat: 18g
- Sodium: 400mg

Number of Servings: 6

Cooking Time: 8 hours 30 minutes

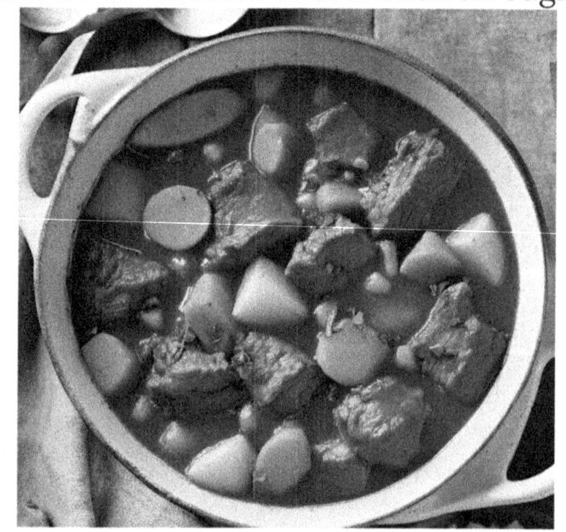

2. Grilled Sirloin Steak

Ingredients:

- 4 (6 oz) sirloin steaks
- 2 tablespoons olive oil
- 2 tablespoons balsamic vinegar
- 1 teaspoon garlic powder
- 1 teaspoon dried rosemary

Instructions:

1. Preheat the grill to medium-high heat.
2. In a small bowl, mix the olive oil, balsamic vinegar, garlic powder, and dried rosemary.
3. Brush the steaks with the olive oil mixture.
4. Grill the steaks for 4-5 minutes per side for medium-rare, or until the desired doneness is reached.
5. Remove from the grill and let rest for 5 minutes before serving.

Nutrition Info (per serving):

- Calories: 320
- Protein: 28g
- Carbohydrates: 2g
- Fiber: 0g
- Sugars: 0g
- Fat: 22g
- Sodium: 100mg

Number of Servings: 4
Cooking Time: 15 minutes

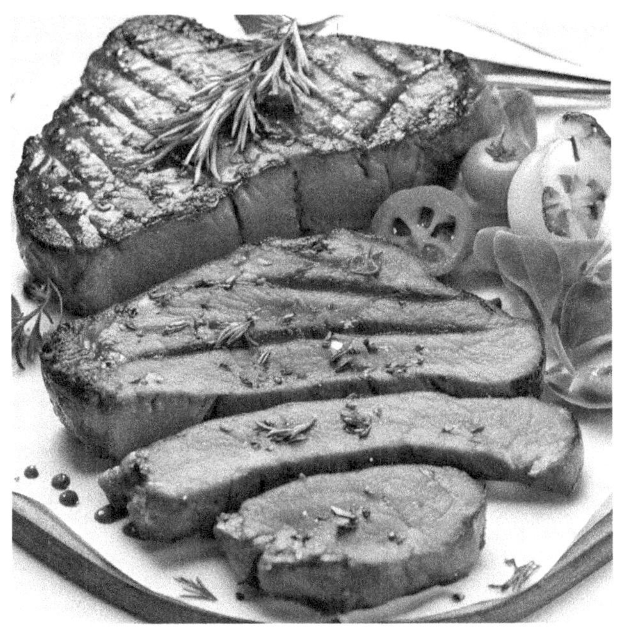

3. Beef and Broccoli Stir-Fry

Ingredients:

- 1 lb beef flank steak, thinly sliced
- 2 tablespoons olive oil
- 3 garlic cloves, minced
- 1 tablespoon grated ginger
- 1 head broccoli, cut into florets
- 1 red bell pepper, sliced
- 1/4 cup low-sodium soy sauce
- 1 tablespoon honey
- 1 tablespoon cornstarch mixed with 2 tablespoons water
- 2 tablespoons chopped green onions

Instructions:

1. Heat olive oil in a large skillet or wok over medium-high heat.
2. Add the garlic and ginger, and cook for 1-2 minutes until fragrant.
3. Add the beef slices and cook until browned, about 5-7 minutes.
4. Remove the beef from the skillet and set aside.
5. In the same skillet, add the broccoli and red bell pepper. Stir-fry for 5-6 minutes until the vegetables are tender-crisp.
6. Return the beef to the skillet.
7. In a small bowl, mix soy sauce, honey, and cornstarch mixture. Pour over the beef and vegetables, stirring to coat evenly.
8. Cook for another 2-3 minutes until the sauce thickens.
9. Sprinkle with chopped green onions and serve immediately.

Nutrition Info (per serving):

- Calories: 300
- Protein: 28g
- Carbohydrates: 14g
- Fiber: 4g
- Sugars: 6g
- Fat: 16g
- Sodium: 500mg

Number of Servings: 4

Cooking Time: 20 minutes

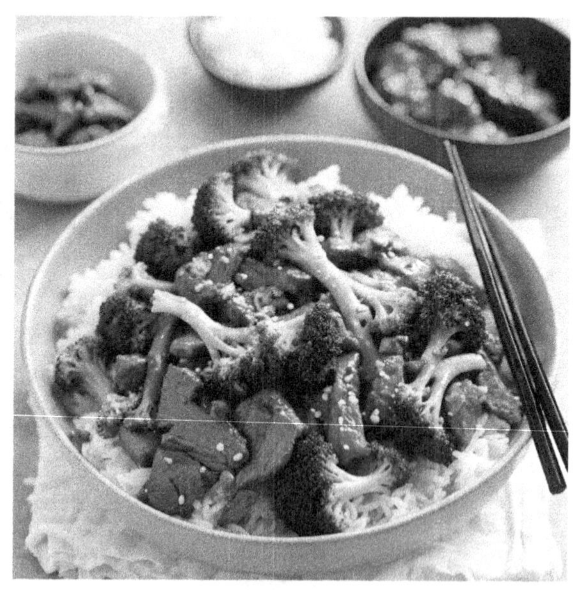

4. Balsamic Glazed Beef Roast

Ingredients:

- 3 lbs beef chuck roast
- 2 tablespoons olive oil
- 1/2 cup balsamic vinegar
- 1/4 cup low-sodium beef broth
- 2 tablespoons honey
- 1 onion, chopped
- 3 garlic cloves, minced
- 1 teaspoon dried thyme

Instructions:

1. Preheat the oven to 350°F (175°C).
2. Heat olive oil in a large oven-safe skillet over medium-high heat.
3. Add the beef roast and sear on all sides until browned, about 4-5 minutes per side.
4. Remove the beef from the skillet and set aside.
5. In the same skillet, add the chopped onion and minced garlic. Cook for 3-4 minutes until softened.
6. Stir in the balsamic vinegar, beef broth, honey, and dried thyme. Bring to a simmer.
7. Return the beef to the skillet and spoon some of the glaze over the top.
8. Cover the skillet and transfer to the oven. Roast for 2-3 hours, or until the beef is tender.
9. Let the roast rest for 10 minutes before slicing and serving with the glaze.

Nutrition Info (per serving):

- Calories: 350
- Protein: 30g
- Carbohydrates: 10g
- Fiber: 1g
- Sugars: 8g
- Fat: 20g
- Sodium: 200mg

Number of Servings: 6
Cooking Time: 3 hours 15 minutes

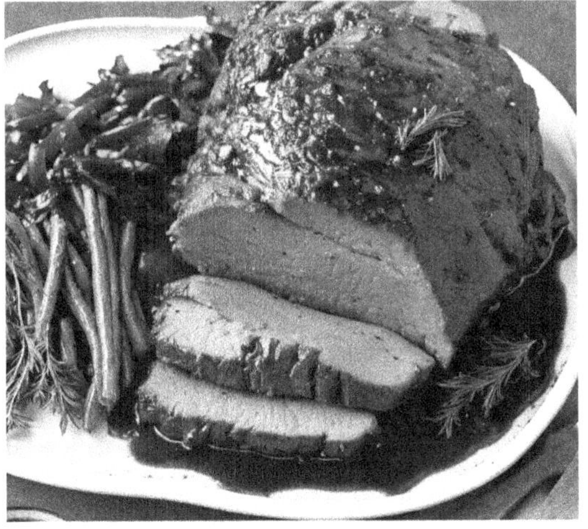

5. Grilled Pork Tenderloin

Ingredients:

- 2 pork tenderloins (about 1 lb each)
- 2 tablespoons olive oil
- 1 tablespoon Dijon mustard
- 1 tablespoon honey
- 1 teaspoon garlic powder
- 1 teaspoon dried thyme

Instructions:

1. Preheat the grill to medium-high heat.
2. In a small bowl, mix the olive oil, Dijon mustard, honey, garlic powder, and dried thyme.
3. Brush the pork tenderloins with the olive oil mixture.
4. Grill the pork tenderloins for 15-20 minutes, turning occasionally, until the internal temperature reaches 145°F (63°C).
5. Remove from the grill and let rest for 5 minutes before slicing.
6. Serve immediately.

Nutrition Info (per serving):

- Calories: 250
- Protein: 28g
- Carbohydrates: 4g
- Fiber: 0g
- Sugars: 3g
- Fat: 12g
- Sodium: 100mg

Number of Servings: 4
Cooking Time: 25 minutes

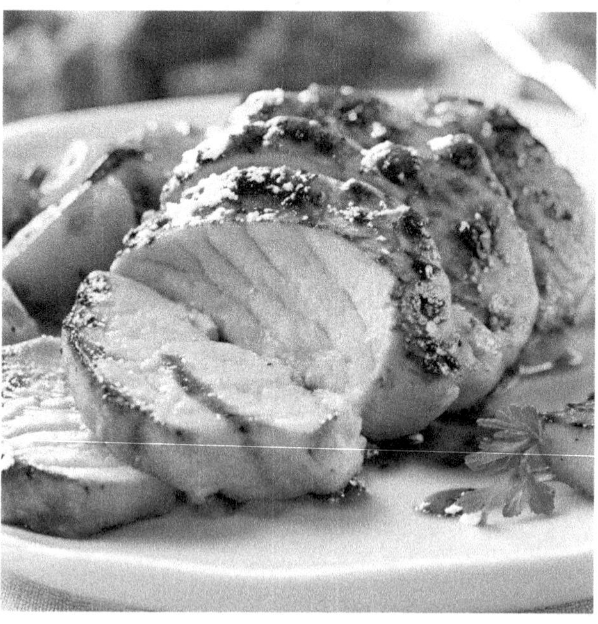

6. Pork and Apple Stew

Ingredients:

- 2 lbs pork shoulder, cut into 1-inch cubes
- 2 tablespoons olive oil
- 1 onion, chopped
- 2 carrots, sliced
- 2 apples, peeled and diced
- 3 garlic cloves, minced
- 4 cups low-sodium chicken broth
- 1 cup apple cider
- 1 teaspoon dried thyme
- 1 teaspoon ground cinnamon
- 1/4 cup chopped fresh parsley

Instructions:

1. Heat olive oil in a large pot over medium heat. Add the pork cubes and brown on all sides, about 5-7 minutes.
2. Add the chopped onion, carrots, and minced garlic to the pot. Cook for 3-4 minutes until the vegetables are softened.
3. Stir in the chicken broth, apple cider, dried thyme, and ground cinnamon. Bring to a boil.
4. Reduce heat and simmer for 1 hour, or until the pork is tender.
5. Add the diced apples and cook for another 15-20 minutes until the apples are tender.
6. Stir in the chopped fresh parsley and serve hot.

Nutrition Info (per serving):

- Calories: 320
- Protein: 28g
- Carbohydrates: 20g
- Fiber: 4g
- Sugars: 12g
- Fat: 14g
- Sodium: 400mg

Number of Servings: 6

Cooking Time: 1 hour 30 minutes

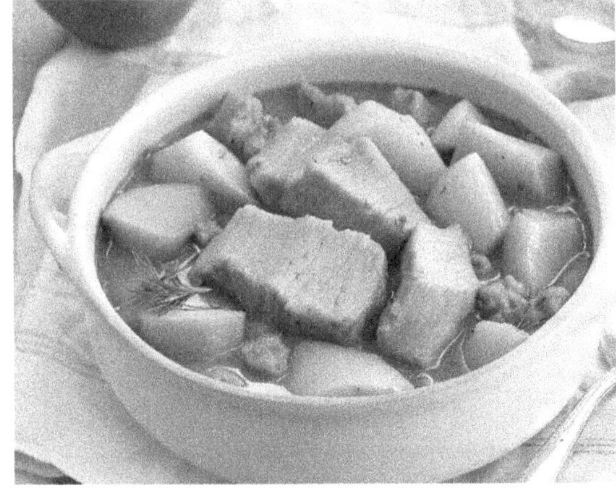

7. Pork Chops with Peach Salsa

Ingredients:

- 4 boneless pork chops (about 6 oz each)
- 2 tablespoons olive oil
- 1 teaspoon garlic powder
- 1 teaspoon dried thyme
- 2 cups diced peaches (fresh or canned)
- 1/4 cup red onion, finely chopped
- 1 jalapeno, seeded and finely chopped
- 1 tablespoon lime juice
- 2 tablespoons chopped fresh cilantro

Instructions:

1. Preheat the grill to medium-high heat.
2. In a small bowl, mix the olive oil, garlic powder, and dried thyme.
3. Brush the pork chops with the olive oil mixture.
4. Grill the pork chops for 4-5 minutes per side, or until the internal temperature reaches 145°F (63°C).
5. Remove from the grill and let rest for 5 minutes.
6. In a medium bowl, combine the diced peaches, red onion, jalapeno, lime juice, and chopped fresh cilantro. Mix well.
7. Serve the pork chops topped with peach salsa.

Nutrition Info (per serving):

- Calories: 300
- Protein: 28g
- Carbohydrates: 12g
- Fiber: 2g
- Sugars: 9g
- Fat: 14g
- Sodium: 200mg

Number of Servings: 4

Cooking Time: 15 minutes

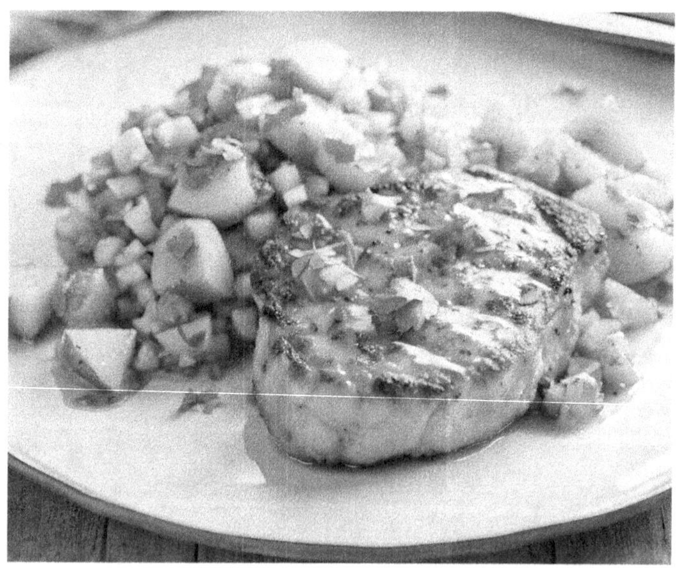

8. Stir-Fried Pork with Ginger and Honey

Ingredients:

- 1 lb pork tenderloin, thinly sliced
- 2 tablespoons olive oil
- 3 garlic cloves, minced
- 1 tablespoon grated ginger
- 1 red bell pepper, sliced
- 1 yellow bell pepper, sliced
- 1 cup snap peas
- 1/4 cup low-sodium soy sauce
- 2 tablespoons honey
- 1 tablespoon rice vinegar
- 1 tablespoon cornstarch mixed with 2 tablespoons water

Instructions:

1. Heat olive oil in a large skillet or wok over medium-high heat.
2. Add the garlic and ginger, and cook for 1-2 minutes until fragrant.
3. Add the pork slices and cook until browned, about 5-7 minutes.
4. Remove the pork from the skillet and set aside.
5. In the same skillet, add the red bell pepper, yellow bell pepper, and snap peas. Stir-fry for 5-6 minutes until the vegetables are tender-crisp.
6. Return the pork to the skillet.
7. In a small bowl, mix soy sauce, honey, rice vinegar, and cornstarch mixture. Pour over the pork and vegetables, stirring to coat evenly.
8. Cook for another 2-3 minutes until the sauce thickens.
9. Scrve immediately.

Nutrition Info (per serving):

- Calories: 280
- Protein: 26g
- Carbohydrates: 16g
- Fiber: 3g
- Sugars: 10g
- Fat: 12g
- Sodium: 500mg

Number of Servings: 4
Cooking Time: 20 minutes

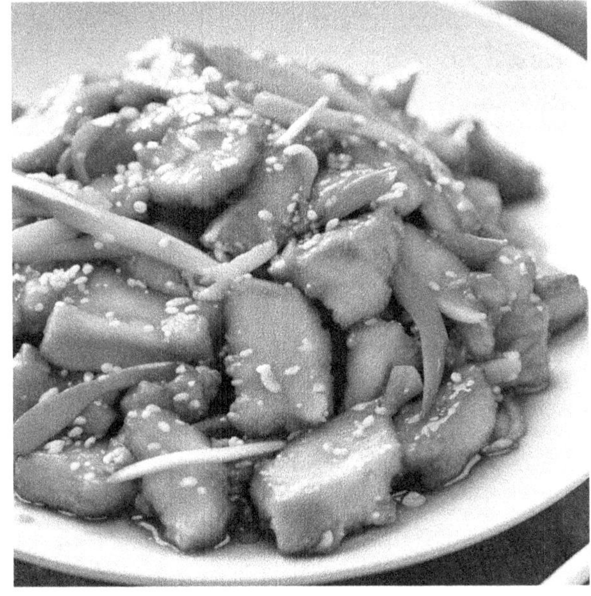

9. Beef Goulash

Ingredients:

- 2 lbs beef chuck, cut into 1-inch cubes
- 2 tablespoons olive oil
- 1 onion, chopped
- 2 garlic cloves, minced
- 1 red bell pepper, chopped
- 1 yellow bell pepper, chopped
- 3 tablespoons paprika
- 1 teaspoon caraway seeds
- 4 cups low-sodium beef broth
- 1 can (14.5 oz) diced tomatoes
- 2 tablespoons tomato paste
- 3 carrots, sliced
- 3 potatoes, diced
- 1/4 cup chopped fresh parsley

Instructions:

1. Heat olive oil in a large pot over medium heat. Add beef and brown on all sides, about 5-7 minutes.
2. Add onion, garlic, and bell peppers. Cook for 3-4 minutes until softened.
3. Stir in paprika and caraway seeds, and cook for another 1-2 minutes.
4. Add beef broth, diced tomatoes, and tomato paste. Bring to a simmer.
5. Add carrots and potatoes. Cover and simmer for 1 1/2 to 2 hours, or until the beef is tender.
6. Garnish with chopped fresh parsley and serve.

Nutrition Info (per serving):

- Calories: 350
- Protein: 28g
- Carbohydrates: 30g
- Fiber: 6g
- Sugars: 8g
- Fat: 14g
- Sodium: 450mg

Number of Servings: 6

Cooking Time: 2 hours 15 minutes

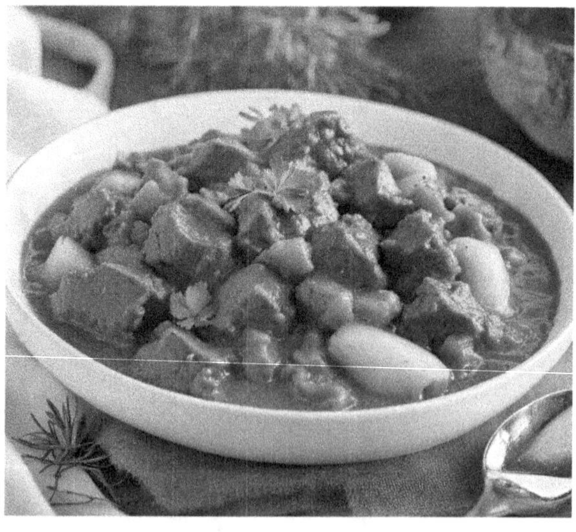

10. Beef Barley Soup

Ingredients:

- 1 lb beef stew meat, cut into 1-inch cubes
- 2 tablespoons olive oil
- 1 onion, chopped
- 2 garlic cloves, minced
- 3 carrots, sliced
- 2 celery stalks, sliced
- 8 cups low-sodium beef broth
- 1/2 cup pearl barley
- 1 teaspoon dried thyme
- 1/2 teaspoon ground black pepper
- 1 cup mushrooms, sliced
- 1/4 cup chopped fresh parsley

Instructions:

1. Heat olive oil in a large pot over medium heat. Add beef and brown on all sides, about 5-7 minutes.
2. Add onion, garlic, carrots, and celery. Cook for 5-7 minutes until the vegetables are tender.
3. Stir in beef broth, barley, dried thyme, and black pepper. Bring to a boil.
4. Reduce heat and simmer for 1 hour, or until the beef and barley are tender.
5. Add mushrooms and cook for another 15 minutes.
6. Stir in chopped fresh parsley and serve.

Nutrition Info (per serving):

- Calories: 280
- Protein: 22g
- Carbohydrates: 28g
- Fiber: 6g
- Sugars: 6g
- Fat: 10g
- Sodium: 400mg

Number of Servings: 6

Cooking Time: 1 hour 30 minutes

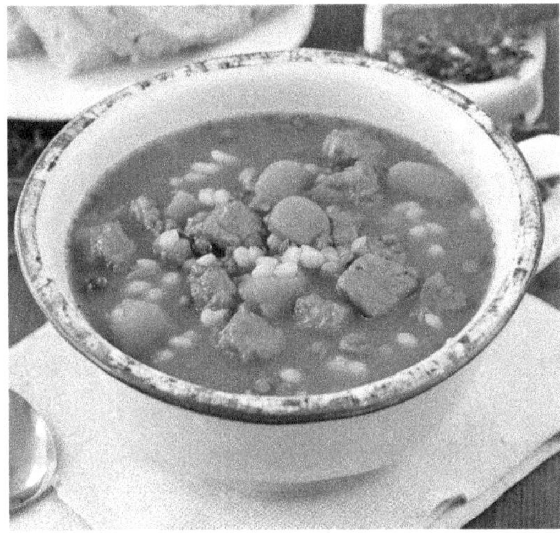

11. Meatloaf with Turkey and Beef

Ingredients:

- 1 lb ground beef
- 1 lb ground turkey
- 1 cup breadcrumbs
- 1 onion, finely chopped
- 2 garlic cloves, minced
- 1/2 cup milk
- 1 egg, beaten
- 2 tablespoons Worcestershire sauce
- 1 teaspoon dried thyme
- 1/2 teaspoon ground black pepper
- 1/4 cup ketchup

Instructions:

1. Preheat the oven to 375°F (190°C).
2. In a large bowl, combine ground beef, ground turkey, breadcrumbs, chopped onion, minced garlic, milk, beaten egg, Worcestershire sauce, dried thyme, and black pepper. Mix until well combined.
3. Shape the mixture into a loaf and place it in a baking dish.
4. Spread ketchup evenly over the top of the meatloaf.
5. Bake for 1 hour, or until the internal temperature reaches 165°F (74°C).
6. Let rest for 10 minutes before slicing and serving.

Nutrition Info (per serving):

- Calories: 320
- Protein: 28g
- Carbohydrates: 15g
- Fiber: 2g
- Sugars: 5g
- Fat: 16g
- Sodium: 350mg

Number of Servings: 6
Cooking Time: 1 hour 20 minutes

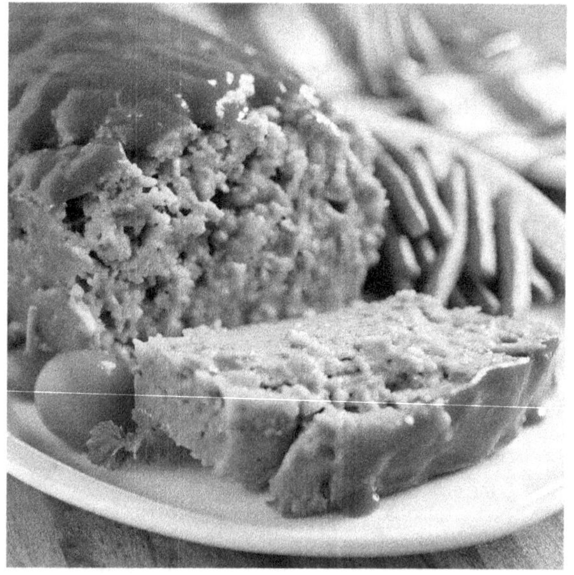

12. Italian Beef Ragu

Ingredients:

- 2 lbs beef chuck, cut into 1-inch cubes
- 2 tablespoons olive oil
- 1 onion, chopped
- 3 garlic cloves, minced
- 1 carrot, finely chopped
- 1 celery stalk, finely chopped
- 1 cup red wine
- 1 can (28 oz) crushed tomatoes
- 1 tablespoon tomato paste
- 1 teaspoon dried basil
- 1 teaspoon dried oregano
- 1/2 teaspoon ground black pepper
- 1/4 cup chopped fresh basil
- 1/4 cup grated Parmesan cheese (optional, for serving)

Instructions:

1. Heat olive oil in a large pot over medium heat. Add beef and brown on all sides, about 5-7 minutes.
2. Add onion, garlic, carrot, and celery. Cook for 5-7 minutes until the vegetables are tender.
3. Stir in red wine, crushed tomatoes, tomato paste, dried basil, dried oregano, and black pepper. Bring to a simmer.
4. Cover and cook on low heat for 2-3 hours, or until the beef is tender.
5. Stir in chopped fresh basil before serving.
6. Serve with grated Parmesan cheese if desired.

Nutrition Info (per serving):

- Calories: 350
- Protein: 28g
- Carbohydrates: 12g
- Fiber: 4g
- Sugars: 6g
- Fat: 18g
- Sodium: 350mg

Number of Servings: 6

Cooking Time: 3 hours 15 minutes

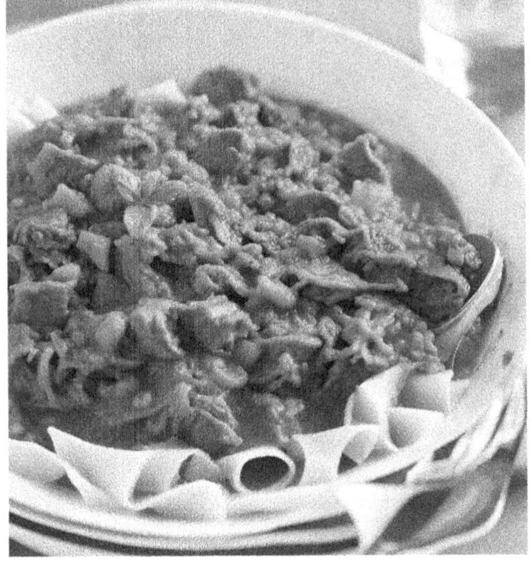

13. Beef Carpaccio

Ingredients:

- 1 lb beef tenderloin
- 2 tablespoons olive oil
- 2 tablespoons lemon juice
- 1 teaspoon Dijon mustard
- 1 cup arugula
- 1/4 cup shaved Parmesan cheese
- 2 tablespoons capers
- 1/4 teaspoon ground black pepper

Instructions:

1. Wrap the beef tenderloin in plastic wrap and freeze for 1 hour to firm up.
2. Using a sharp knife, thinly slice the beef.
3. Arrange the beef slices on a large platter.
4. In a small bowl, whisk together olive oil, lemon juice, and Dijon mustard.
5. Drizzle the dressing over the beef slices.
6. Top with arugula, shaved Parmesan cheese, capers, and ground black pepper.
7. Serve immediately.

Nutrition Info (per serving):

- Calories: 250
- Protein: 26g
- Carbohydrates: 2g
- Fiber: 1g
- Sugars: 0g
- Fat: 16g
- Sodium: 200mg

Number of Servings: 4
Cooking Time: 10 minutes

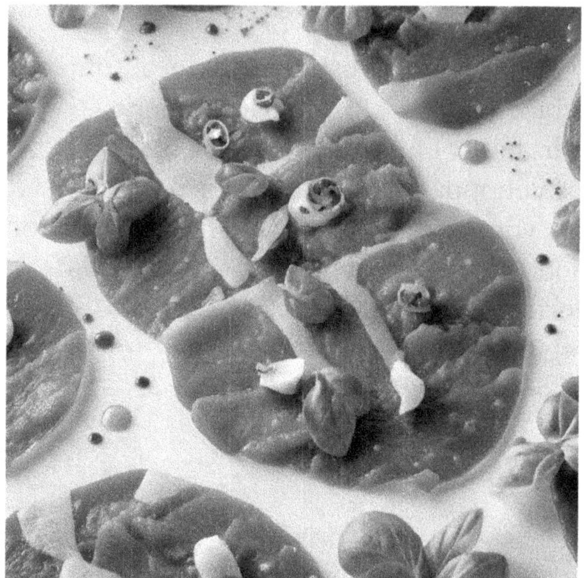

14. Thai Beef Salad

Ingredients:

- 1 lb beef sirloin, thinly sliced
- 2 tablespoons olive oil
- 1 tablespoon fish sauce
- 2 tablespoons lime juice
- 1 tablespoon soy sauce
- 1 tablespoon honey
- 1 garlic clove, minced
- 1 cup mixed salad greens
- 1/2 cucumber, sliced
- 1/2 red onion, thinly sliced
- 1/2 cup cherry tomatoes, halved
- 1/4 cup fresh cilantro, chopped
- 1/4 cup fresh mint, chopped
- 1/4 teaspoon red pepper flakes

Instructions:

1. Heat olive oil in a large skillet over medium-high heat. Add the beef slices and cook until browned, about 5-7 minutes. Remove from heat and set aside.
2. In a small bowl, mix fish sauce, lime juice, soy sauce, honey, and minced garlic.
3. In a large bowl, combine mixed salad greens, cucumber, red onion, cherry tomatoes, fresh cilantro, and fresh mint.
4. Add the cooked beef to the salad and toss to combine.
5. Drizzle with the dressing and sprinkle with red pepper flakes.
6. Serve immediately.

Nutrition Info (per serving):

- Calories: 300
- Protein: 26g
- Carbohydrates: 10g
- Fiber: 2g
- Sugars: 6g
- Fat: 18g
- Sodium: 500mg

Number of Servings: 4
Cooking Time: 20 minutes

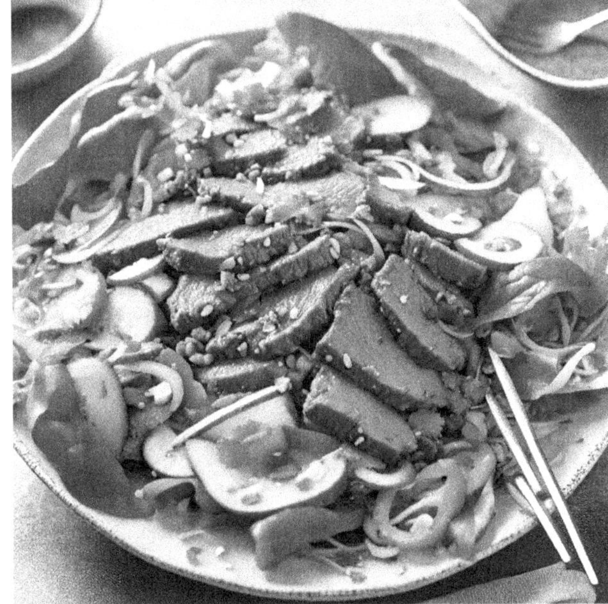

15. Beef Vegetable Pot Pie

Ingredients:

- 1 lb beef stew meat, cut into 1-inch cubes
- 2 tablespoons olive oil
- 1 onion, chopped
- 2 garlic cloves, minced
- 2 carrots, sliced
- 2 celery stalks, sliced
- 1 cup frozen peas
- 1 cup frozen corn
- 2 cups low-sodium beef broth
- 1/2 cup milk
- 1/4 cup all-purpose flour
- 1 teaspoon dried thyme
- 1/2 teaspoon ground black pepper
- 1 sheet puff pastry, thawed

Instructions:

1. Preheat the oven to 400°F (200°C).
2. Heat olive oil in a large skillet over medium heat. Add beef and brown on all sides, about 5-7 minutes.
3. Add onion, garlic, carrots, and celery. Cook for 5-7 minutes until the vegetables are tender.
4. Stir in beef broth, milk, dried thyme, and black pepper.
5. Sprinkle the flour over the mixture and stir until the sauce thickens.
6. Add frozen peas and corn, and cook for another 2-3 minutes.
7. Pour the mixture into a baking dish and cover with the puff pastry sheet, trimming any excess.
8. Bake for 20-25 minutes, or until the pastry is golden brown.
9. Serve immediately.

Nutrition Info (per serving):

- Calories: 400
- Protein: 28g
- Carbohydrates: 35g
- Fiber: 5g
- Sugars: 6g
- Fat: 16g
- Sodium: 450mg

Number of Servings: 6
Cooking Time: 45 minutes

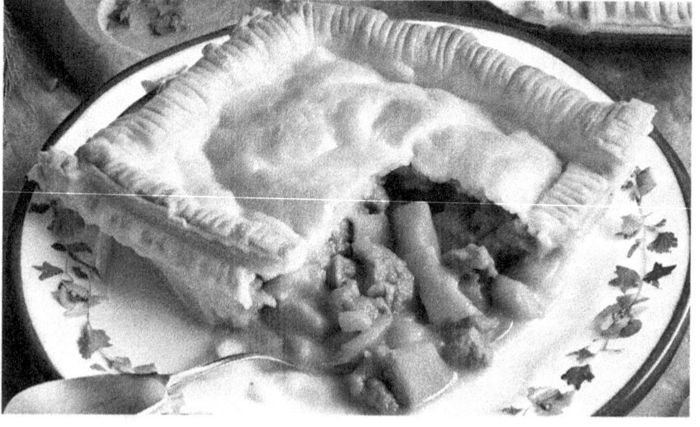

16. Swedish Meatballs

Ingredients:

- 1 lb ground beef
- 1/2 cup breadcrumbs
- 1/4 cup milk
- 1 egg, beaten
- 1 onion, finely chopped
- 1/2 teaspoon ground allspice
- 1/2 teaspoon ground nutmeg
- 2 tablespoons olive oil
- 2 cups low-sodium beef broth
- 1/2 cup heavy cream
- 1 tablespoon Dijon mustard
- 1 tablespoon cornstarch mixed with 2 tablespoons water

Instructions:

1. In a large bowl, combine ground beef, breadcrumbs, milk, beaten egg, chopped onion, ground allspice, and ground nutmeg. Mix until well combined and form into meatballs.
2. Heat olive oil in a large skillet over medium heat. Add the meatballs and cook until browned on all sides, about 5-7 minutes.
3. Remove the meatballs from the skillet and set aside.
4. In the same skillet, add beef broth, heavy cream, and Dijon mustard. Bring to a simmer.
5. Stir in the cornstarch mixture and cook for another 2-3 minutes until the sauce thickens.
6. Return the meatballs to the skillet and cook for another 5 minutes.
7. Serve the meatballs with the sauce.

Nutrition Info (per serving):

- Calories: 350
- Protein: 22g
- Carbohydrates: 12g
- Fiber: 1g
- Sugars: 3g
- Fat: 26g
- Sodium: 450mg

Number of Servings: 4
Cooking Time: 30 minutes

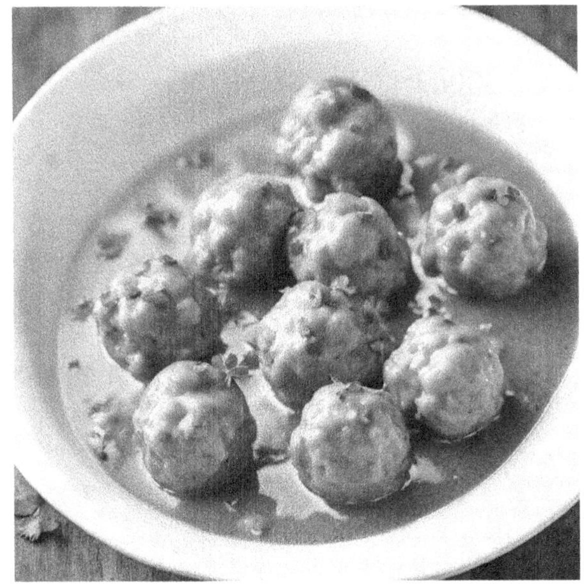

17. Beef and Mushroom Skillet

Ingredients:

- 1 lb beef sirloin, thinly sliced
- 2 tablespoons olive oil
- 1 onion, chopped
- 2 garlic cloves, minced
- 2 cups mushrooms, sliced
- 1/2 cup beef broth
- 1/4 cup red wine (optional)
- 1 teaspoon dried thyme
- 1/2 teaspoon ground black pepper
- 2 tablespoons chopped fresh parsley

Instructions:

1. Heat olive oil in a large skillet over medium-high heat. Add the beef slices and cook until browned, about 5-7 minutes. Remove from heat and set aside.
2. In the same skillet, add the chopped onion and minced garlic. Cook for 3-4 minutes until softened.
3. Add the mushrooms and cook for another 5 minutes.
4. Stir in the beef broth, red wine (if using), dried thyme, and black pepper. Bring to a simmer.
5. Return the beef to the skillet and cook for another 5 minutes.
6. Sprinkle with chopped fresh parsley and serve immediately.

Nutrition Info (per serving):

- Calories: 300
- Protein: 26g
- Carbohydrates: 8g
- Fiber: 2g
- Sugars: 4g
- Fat: 18g
- Sodium: 300mg

Number of Servings: 4
Cooking Time: 25 minutes

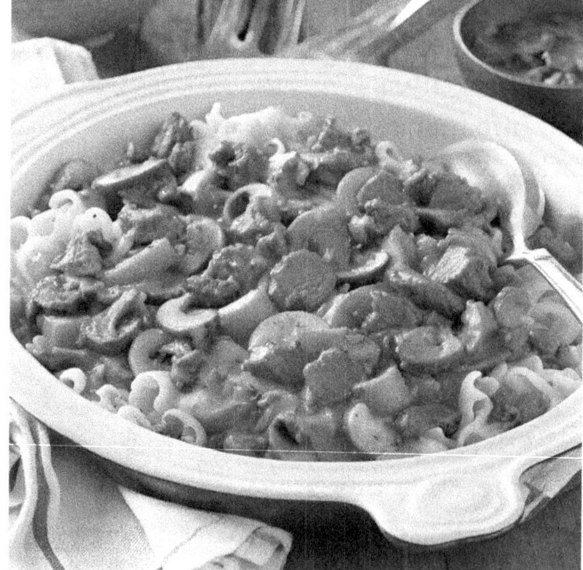

18. Pulled Pork with BBQ Sauce

Ingredients:

- 3 lbs pork shoulder
- 1 tablespoon olive oil
- 1 onion, chopped
- 3 garlic cloves, minced
- 1 cup low-sodium chicken broth
- 1 cup BBQ sauce (homemade or store-bought)
- 1/4 cup apple cider vinegar
- 1 tablespoon brown sugar
- 1 teaspoon smoked paprika
- 1/2 teaspoon ground black pepper

Instructions:

1. Heat olive oil in a large skillet over medium heat. Add the pork shoulder and brown on all sides, about 5-7 minutes.
2. Transfer the pork to a slow cooker.
3. In the same skillet, add the chopped onion and minced garlic. Cook for 3-4 minutes until softened.
4. Add chicken broth, BBQ sauce, apple cider vinegar, brown sugar, smoked paprika, and black pepper. Bring to a simmer.
5. Pour the sauce over the pork in the slow cooker.
6. Cover and cook on low for 8-10 hours, or until the pork is tender and can be easily shredded with a fork.
7. Shred the pork and mix with the sauce.
8. Serve immediately.

Nutrition Info (per serving):

- Calories: 400
- Protein: 28g
- Carbohydrates: 20g
- Fiber: 2g
- Sugars: 12g
- Fat: 24g
- Sodium: 450mg

Number of Servings: 6
Cooking Time: 8 hours 20 minute

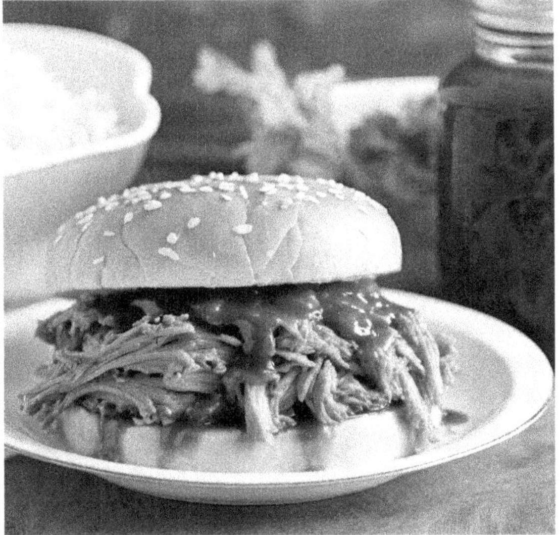

19. Pork Loin Roast with Herbs

Ingredients:

- 2 lbs pork loin roast
- 2 tablespoons olive oil
- 2 garlic cloves, minced
- 1 tablespoon chopped fresh rosemary
- 1 tablespoon chopped fresh thyme
- 1 tablespoon Dijon mustard
- 1/4 teaspoon ground black pepper

Instructions:

1. Preheat the oven to 375°F (190°C).
2. In a small bowl, mix olive oil, minced garlic, chopped rosemary, chopped thyme, Dijon mustard, and black pepper.
3. Rub the mixture all over the pork loin roast.
4. Place the pork in a roasting pan and roast for 1 hour, or until the internal temperature reaches 145°F (63°C).
5. Let the pork rest for 10 minutes before slicing and serving.

Nutrition Info (per serving):

- Calories: 280
- Protein: 28g
- Carbohydrates: 2g
- Fiber: 0g
- Sugars: 0g
- Fat: 18g
- Sodium: 150mg

Number of Servings: 6

Cooking Time: 1 hour 10 minutes

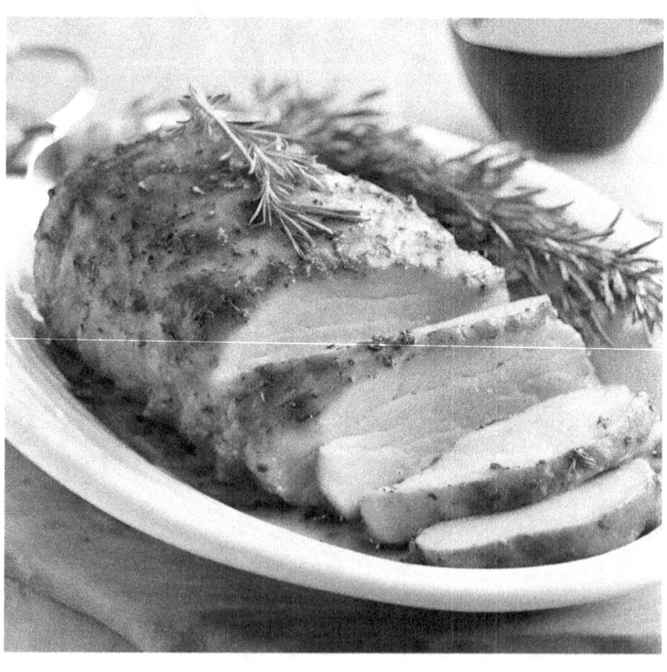

20. Pork and Pepper Stir-Fry

Ingredients:

- 1 lb pork tenderloin, thinly sliced
- 2 tablespoons olive oil
- 2 garlic cloves, minced
- 1 tablespoon grated ginger
- 1 red bell pepper, sliced
- 1 green bell pepper, sliced
- 1 yellow bell pepper, sliced
- 1/4 cup low-sodium soy sauce
- 1 tablespoon honey
- 1 tablespoon rice vinegar
- 1 tablespoon cornstarch mixed with 2 tablespoons water

Instructions:

1. Heat olive oil in a large skillet or wok over medium-high heat.
2. Add the garlic and ginger, and cook for 1-2 minutes until fragrant.
3. Add the pork slices and cook until browned, about 5-7 minutes.
4. Remove the pork from the skillet and set aside.
5. In the same skillet, add the red, green, and yellow bell peppers. Stir-fry for 5-6 minutes until the vegetables are tender-crisp.
6. Return the pork to the skillet.
7. In a small bowl, mix soy sauce, honey, rice vinegar, and cornstarch mixture. Pour over the pork and vegetables, stirring to coat evenly.
8. Cook for another 2-3 minutes until the sauce thickens.
9. Serve immediately.

Nutrition Info (per serving):

- Calories: 280
- Protein: 26g
- Carbohydrates: 16g
- Fiber: 3g
- Sugars: 10g
- Fat: 12g
- Sodium: 500mg

Number of Servings: 4

Cooking Time: 20 minutes

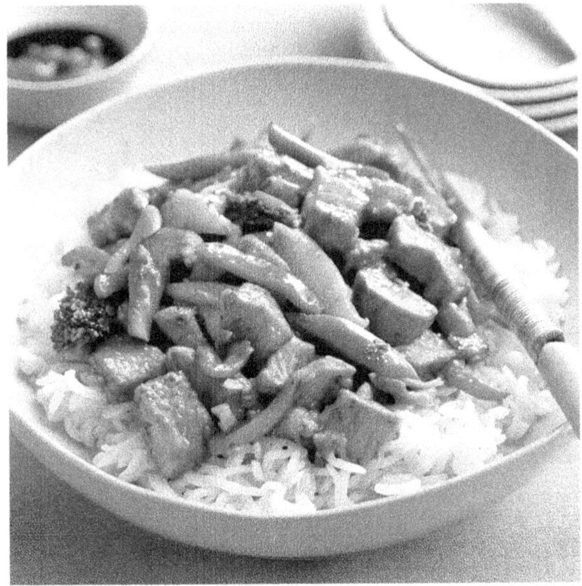

21. Vietnamese Pork Bowls

Ingredients:

- 1 lb ground pork
- 2 tablespoons olive oil
- 1 onion, chopped
- 2 garlic cloves, minced
- 1 tablespoon grated ginger
- 1/4 cup fish sauce
- 2 tablespoons lime juice
- 1 tablespoon honey
- 1 cup cooked rice noodles
- 1 cup shredded carrots
- 1 cup shredded cabbage
- 1/2 cup chopped fresh mint
- 1/4 cup chopped fresh cilantro
- 1/4 cup chopped peanuts

Instructions:

1. Heat olive oil in a large skillet over medium heat. Add chopped onion, minced garlic, and grated ginger. Cook for 3-4 minutes until the onion is soft.
2. Add the ground pork and cook until browned, about 5-7 minutes.
3. Stir in fish sauce, lime juice, and honey. Cook for another 2-3 minutes until the pork is well coated and heated through.
4. Divide the cooked rice noodles among bowls.
5. Top with the pork mixture, shredded carrots, shredded cabbage, fresh mint, fresh cilantro, and chopped peanuts.
6. Serve immediately.

Nutrition Info (per serving):

- Calories: 350
- Protein: 20g
- Carbohydrates: 24g
- Fiber: 3g
- Sugars: 8g
- Fat: 20g
- Sodium: 650mg

Number of Servings: 4
Cooking Time: 20 minutes

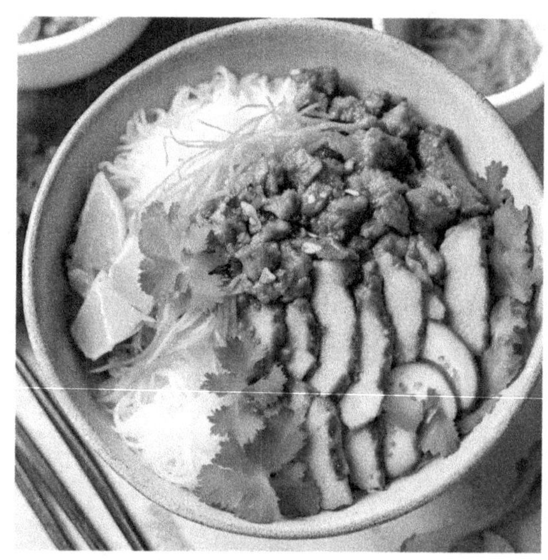

22. Smoky Pork and Bean Soup

Ingredients:

- 1 lb smoked pork sausage, sliced
- 2 tablespoons olive oil
- 1 onion, chopped
- 3 garlic cloves, minced
- 2 carrots, sliced
- 2 celery stalks, sliced
- 4 cups low-sodium chicken broth
- 1 can (14.5 oz) diced tomatoes
- 2 cans (15 oz each) cannellini beans, drained and rinsed
- 1 teaspoon smoked paprika
- 1/2 teaspoon ground black pepper
- 1/4 cup chopped fresh parsley

Instructions:

1. Heat olive oil in a large pot over medium heat. Add smoked pork sausage and cook until browned, about 5-7 minutes.
2. Add chopped onion, minced garlic, carrots, and celery. Cook for 5-7 minutes until the vegetables are tender.
3. Stir in chicken broth, diced tomatoes, cannellini beans, smoked paprika, and black pepper. Bring to a boil.
4. Reduce heat and simmer for 30 minutes.
5. Stir in chopped fresh parsley and serve.

Nutrition Info (per serving):

- Calories: 350
- Protein: 22g
- Carbohydrates: 24g
- Fiber: 6g
- Sugars: 6g
- Fat: 18g
- Sodium: 600mg

Number of Servings: 6

Cooking Time: 45 minutes

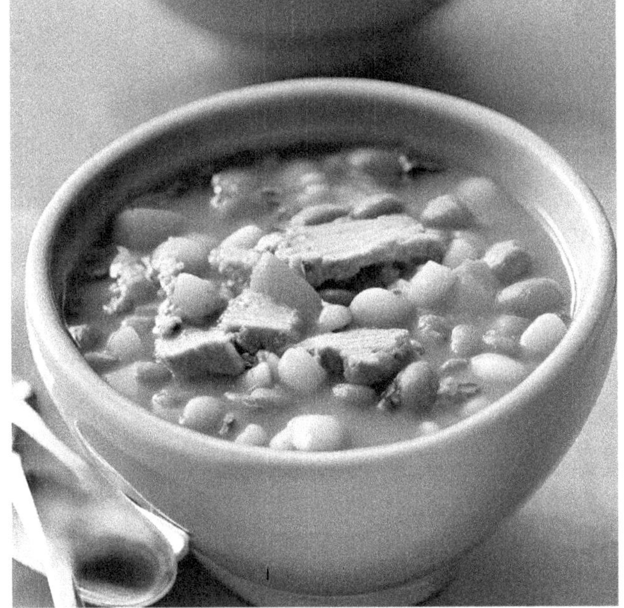

23. Pork Miso Soup

Ingredients:

- 1 lb pork tenderloin, thinly sliced
- 2 tablespoons olive oil
- 1 onion, chopped
- 2 garlic cloves, minced
- 4 cups low-sodium chicken broth
- 1/4 cup miso paste
- 1 cup tofu, cubed
- 1 cup mushrooms, sliced
- 1 cup spinach leaves
- 2 green onions, sliced
- 1 tablespoon soy sauce
- 1 tablespoon rice vinegar

Instructions:

1. Heat olive oil in a large pot over medium heat. Add chopped onion and minced garlic. Cook for 3-4 minutes until softened.
2. Add the pork slices and cook until browned, about 5-7 minutes.
3. Stir in chicken broth, miso paste, and soy sauce. Bring to a simmer.
4. Add tofu, mushrooms, and spinach leaves. Cook for another 5-7 minutes until the vegetables are tender.
5. Stir in rice vinegar and sliced green onions.
6. Serve immediately.

Nutrition Info (per serving):

- Calories: 300
- Protein: 26g
- Carbohydrates: 12g
- Fiber: 2g
- Sugars: 4g
- Fat: 16g
- Sodium: 450mg

Number of Servings: 4
Cooking Time: 20 minutes

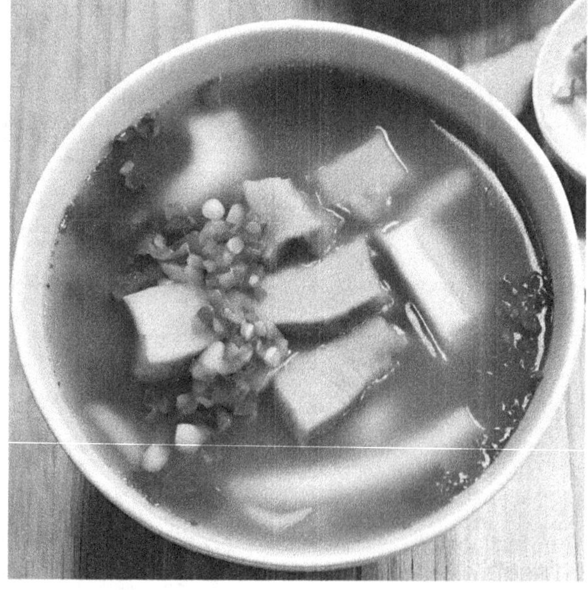

24. German Pork Schnitzel

Ingredients:

- 4 boneless pork chops (about 6 oz each)
- 1/2 cup all-purpose flour
- 2 eggs, beaten
- 1 cup breadcrumbs
- 2 tablespoons olive oil
- 2 tablespoons unsalted butter
- 1 lemon, cut into wedges
- 1/4 cup chopped fresh parsley

Instructions:

1. Pound the pork chops to 1/4-inch thickness.
2. Place the flour, beaten eggs, and breadcrumbs in three separate shallow dishes.
3. Dredge each pork chop in the flour, dip in the beaten eggs, and coat with breadcrumbs.
4. Heat olive oil and unsalted butter in a large skillet over medium heat.
5. Add the pork chops and cook for 3-4 minutes per side, until golden brown and cooked through.
6. Remove from heat and let rest for a few minutes.
7. Serve with lemon wedges and garnish with chopped fresh parsley.

Nutrition Info (per serving):

- Calories: 400
- Protein: 28g
- Carbohydrates: 24g
- Fiber: 2g
- Sugars: 2g
- Fat: 20g
- Sodium: 250mg

Number of Servings: 4
Cooking Time: 20 minutes

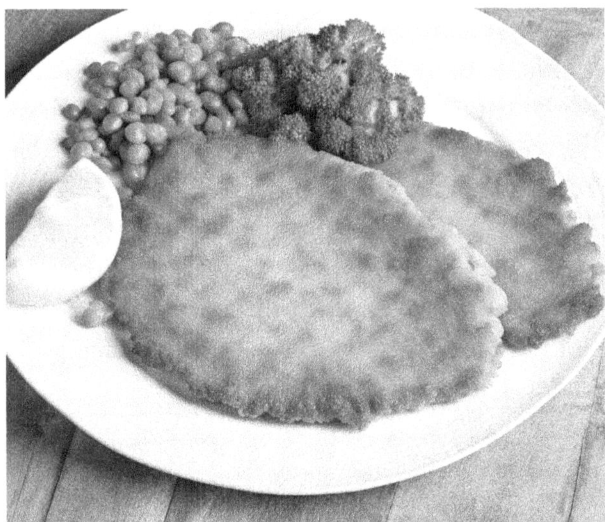

Desserts Recipes

1. Apple Cinnamon Baked Oatmeal Cups
Ingredients:
- 2 cups rolled oats
- 1 teaspoon baking powder
- 1 teaspoon ground cinnamon
- 1/2 teaspoon ground nutmeg
- 1/4 teaspoon ground cloves
- 1/2 cup unsweetened applesauce
- 1 cup almond milk
- 1/4 cup honey
- 1 large egg
- 1 teaspoon vanilla extract
- 1 apple, peeled and diced

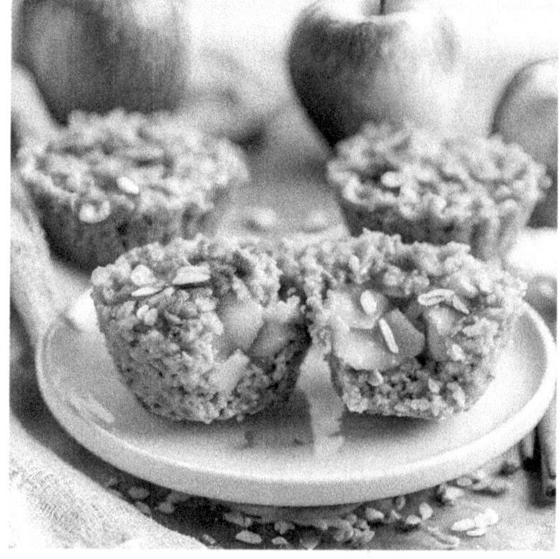

Instructions:
1. Preheat the oven to 350°F (175°C). Grease a 12-cup muffin tin.
2. In a large bowl, mix the rolled oats, baking powder, ground cinnamon, ground nutmeg, and ground cloves.
3. In another bowl, whisk together the applesauce, almond milk, honey, egg, and vanilla extract.
4. Pour the wet ingredients into the dry ingredients and mix until well combined.
5. Fold in the diced apple.
6. Divide the mixture evenly among the muffin cups.
7. Bake for 25-30 minutes, or until the tops are golden and a toothpick inserted into the center comes out clean.
8. Let cool for a few minutes before serving.

Nutrition Info (per serving):
- Calories: 150
- Protein: 3g
- Carbohydrates: 28g
- Fiber: 3g
- Sugars: 12g
- Fat: 3g
- Sodium: 60mg

Number of Servings: 12
Cooking Time: 30 minutes

2. Banana Nut Bread

Ingredients:

- 3 ripe bananas, mashed
- 1/3 cup melted coconut oil
- 1/4 cup honey
- 1 large egg
- 1 teaspoon vanilla extract
- 1 teaspoon baking soda
- 1/2 teaspoon ground cinnamon
- 1 1/2 cups whole wheat flour
- 1/2 cup chopped walnuts

Instructions:

1. Preheat the oven to 350°F (175°C). Grease a 9x5-inch loaf pan.
2. In a large bowl, mix the mashed bananas, melted coconut oil, honey, egg, and vanilla extract.
3. Add the baking soda, ground cinnamon, and whole wheat flour. Stir until just combined.
4. Fold in the chopped walnuts.
5. Pour the batter into the prepared loaf pan.
6. Bake for 50-60 minutes, or until a toothpick inserted into the center comes out clean.
7. Let cool in the pan for 10 minutes before transferring to a wire rack to cool completely.

Nutrition Info (per serving):

- Calories: 200
- Protein: 4g
- Carbohydrates: 30g
- Fiber: 4g
- Sugars: 12g
- Fat: 8g
- Sodium: 130mg

Number of Servings: 10

Cooking Time: 60 minutes

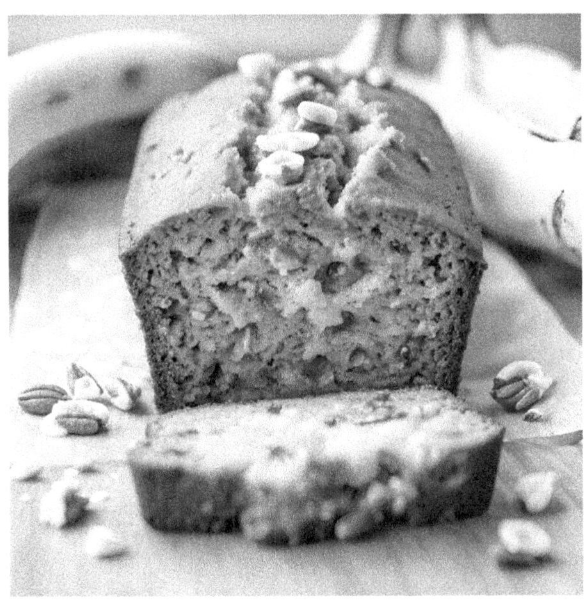

3. Carrot Cake with Cream Cheese Frosting

Ingredients for Cake:

- 2 cups whole wheat flour
- 2 teaspoons baking powder
- 1 1/2 teaspoons ground cinnamon
- 1/2 teaspoon ground nutmeg
- 1/2 teaspoon ground ginger
- 1/4 teaspoon ground cloves
- 3 large eggs
- 1/2 cup coconut oil, melted
- 3/4 cup honey
- 1 teaspoon vanilla extract
- 2 cups grated carrots
- 1/2 cup crushed pineapple, drained
- 1/2 cup chopped walnuts

Ingredients for Frosting:

- 8 oz cream cheese, softened
- 1/4 cup honey
- 1 teaspoon vanilla extract

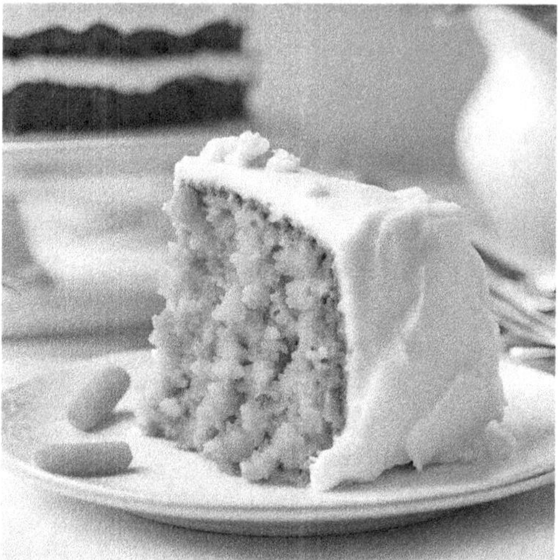

Instructions:

1. Preheat the oven to 350°F (175°C). Grease and flour a 9x13-inch baking pan.
2. In a large bowl, whisk together the flour, baking powder, cinnamon, nutmeg, ginger, and cloves.
3. In another bowl, beat the eggs, melted coconut oil, honey, and vanilla extract until well combined.
4. Add the wet ingredients to the dry ingredients and stir until just combined.
5. Fold in the grated carrots, crushed pineapple, and chopped walnuts.
6. Pour the batter into the prepared pan and spread evenly.
7. Bake for 30-35 minutes, or until a toothpick inserted into the center comes out clean.
8. Let the cake cool completely before frosting.
9. To make the frosting, beat the cream cheese, honey, and vanilla extract until smooth.
10. Spread the frosting over the cooled cake.
11. Cut into squares and serve.

Nutrition Info (per serving):

- Calories: 250   Protein: 5g   Carbohydrates: 30g
- Fiber: 4g
- Sugars: 18g
- Fat: 12g
- Sodium: 150mg

Number of Servings: 12

Cooking Time: 35 minutes

4. Chia Seed Pudding with Berries

Ingredients:

- 1/2 cup chia seeds
- 2 cups almond milk
- 1/4 cup honey
- 1 teaspoon vanilla extract
- 1 cup mixed berries (strawberries, blueberries, raspberries)

Instructions:

1. In a medium bowl, mix the chia seeds, almond milk, honey, and vanilla extract.
2. Stir well to combine and let sit for 5 minutes. Stir again to prevent clumping.
3. Cover and refrigerate for at least 4 hours or overnight.
4. Stir the pudding before serving.
5. Divide the pudding into four bowls and top with mixed berries.

Nutrition Info (per serving):

- Calories: 200
- Protein: 4g
- Carbohydrates: 28g
- Fiber: 9g
- Sugars: 18g
- Fat: 9g
- Sodium: 60mg

Number of Servings: 4
Cooking Time: 4 hours (refrigeration)

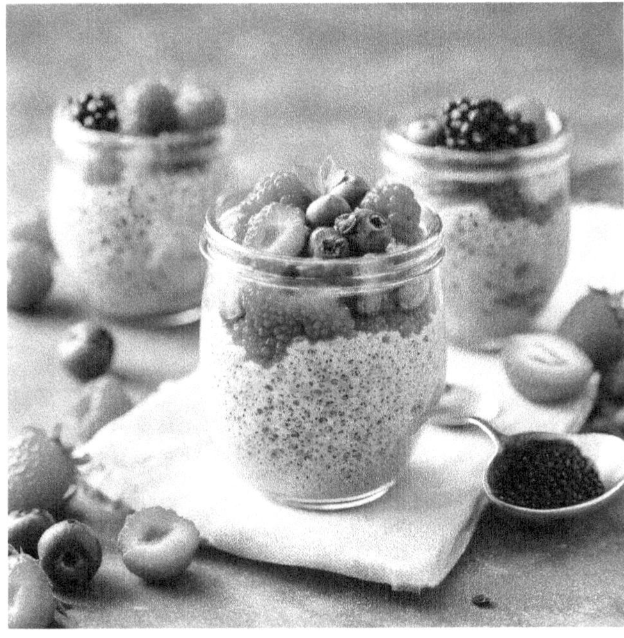

5. Whole Grain Blueberry Muffins

Ingredients:

- 1 1/2 cups whole wheat flour
- 1/2 cup rolled oats
- 1/2 cup honey
- 1 teaspoon baking powder
- 1/2 teaspoon baking soda
- 1 teaspoon ground cinnamon
- 1/2 cup unsweetened applesauce
- 1/2 cup almond milk
- 1 large egg
- 1 teaspoon vanilla extract
- 1 cup fresh or frozen blueberries

Instructions:

1. Preheat the oven to 350°F (175°C). Grease a 12-cup muffin tin or line with paper liners.
2. In a large bowl, mix the flour, oats, baking powder, baking soda, and cinnamon.
3. In another bowl, whisk together the applesauce, almond milk, honey, egg, and vanilla extract.
4. Pour the wet ingredients into the dry ingredients and stir until just combined.
5. Fold in the blueberries.
6. Divide the batter evenly among the muffin cups.
7. Bake for 20-25 minutes, or until a toothpick inserted into the center comes out clean.
8. Let cool for a few minutes before serving.

Nutrition Info (per serving):

- Calories: 150
- Protein: 4g
- Carbohydrates: 30g
- Fiber: 3g
- Sugars: 12g
- Fat: 3g
- Sodium: 100mg

Number of Servings: 12
Cooking Time: 25 minutes

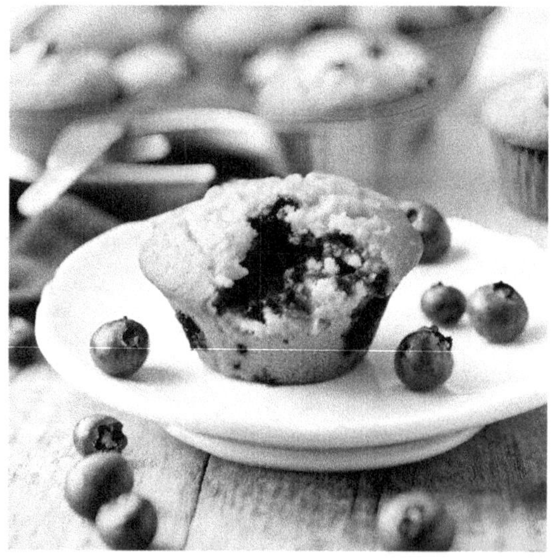

6. Baked Pears with Honey and Walnuts

Ingredients:

- 4 ripe pears, halved and cored
- 1/4 cup honey
- 1 teaspoon ground cinnamon
- 1/4 cup chopped walnuts

Instructions:

1. Preheat the oven to 350°F (175°C). Grease a baking dish.
2. Place the pear halves in the baking dish, cut side up.
3. Drizzle the honey over the pears and sprinkle with cinnamon.
4. Top with chopped walnuts.
5. Bake for 20-25 minutes, or until the pears are tender.
6. Serve warm.

Nutrition Info (per serving):

- Calories: 150
- Protein: 2g
- Carbohydrates: 28g
- Fiber: 4g
- Sugars: 20g
- Fat: 6g
- Sodium: 0mg

Number of Servings: 8

Cooking Time: 25 minutes

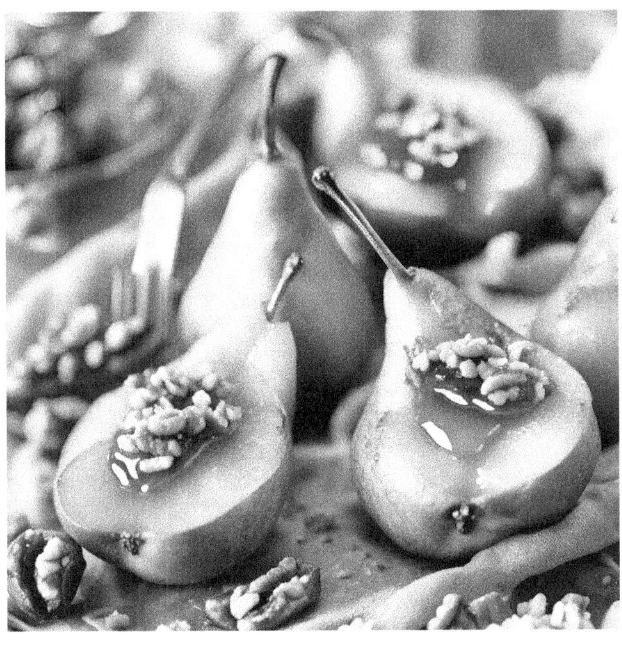

7. No-Bake Chocolate Oat Bars

Ingredients:

- 3 cups rolled oats
- 1 cup peanut butter
- 1/2 cup honey
- 1/2 cup coconut oil
- 1/2 cup dark chocolate chips
- 1 teaspoon vanilla extract

Instructions:

1. In a medium saucepan, combine the peanut butter, honey, and coconut oil. Heat over medium heat until melted and smooth, stirring occasionally.
2. Remove from heat and stir in the vanilla extract and rolled oats until well combined.
3. Press half of the mixture into the bottom of a greased 9x13-inch baking dish.
4. Melt the dark chocolate chips in a microwave-safe bowl in 30-second intervals, stirring in between, until fully melted.
5. Spread the melted chocolate over the oat mixture in the baking dish.
6. Press the remaining oat mixture over the chocolate layer.
7. Refrigerate for at least 2 hours before cutting into bars.
8. Store in the refrigerator.

Nutrition Info (per serving):

- Calories: 200
- Protein: 5g
- Carbohydrates: 20g
- Fiber: 3g
- Sugars: 10g
- Fat: 12g
- Sodium: 50mg

Number of Servings: 16

Cooking Time: 2 hours (refrigeration)

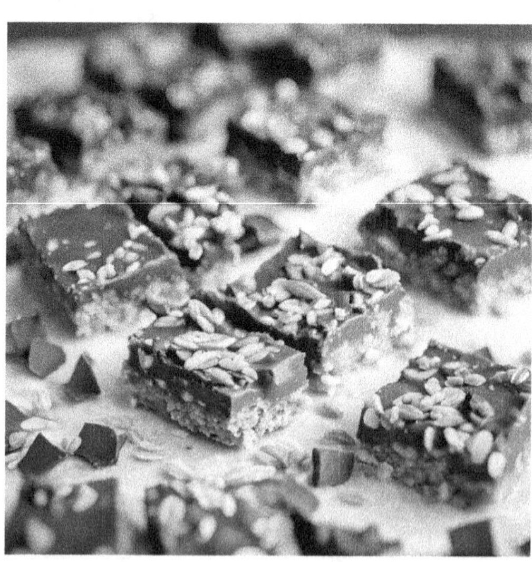

8. Almond and Date Truffles

Ingredients:

- 1 cup pitted dates
- 1 cup almonds
- 1/4 cup unsweetened cocoa powder
- 1 teaspoon vanilla extract
- 1/4 cup shredded coconut (optional)

Instructions:

1. In a food processor, combine the dates and almonds. Process until finely chopped and well mixed.
2. Add the cocoa powder and vanilla extract. Process until the mixture forms a sticky dough.
3. Roll the mixture into small balls.
4. Optional: Roll the balls in shredded coconut to coat.
5. Place the truffles in the refrigerator for at least 30 minutes before serving.
6. Store in the refrigerator.

Nutrition Info (per serving):

- Calories: 120
- Protein: 3g
- Carbohydrates: 18g
- Fiber: 4g
- Sugars: 14g
- Fat: 5g
- Sodium: 0mg

Number of Servings: 16
Cooking Time: 30 minutes (refrigeration)

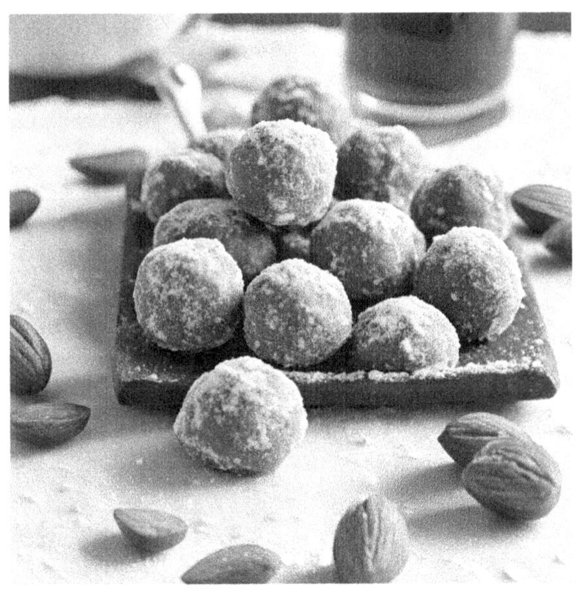

9. Fruit Salad with Citrus Mint Dressing
Ingredients:

- 2 cups strawberries, hulled and quartered
- 2 cups blueberries
- 2 cups pineapple, diced
- 2 kiwis, peeled and sliced
- 1 orange, peeled and segmented
- 1/4 cup fresh mint, chopped
- 1/4 cup orange juice
- 1 tablespoon honey
- 1 teaspoon lime juice

Instructions:

1. In a large bowl, combine the strawberries, blueberries, pineapple, kiwis, and orange segments.
2. In a small bowl, whisk together the orange juice, honey, and lime juice.
3. Pour the dressing over the fruit and toss gently to coat.
4. Sprinkle with chopped fresh mint.
5. Serve immediately or refrigerate until ready to serve.

Nutrition Info (per serving):

- Calories: 80
- Protein: 1g
- Carbohydrates: 20g
- Fiber: 4g
- Sugars: 16g
- Fat: 0g
- Sodium: 5mg

Number of Servings: 8
Cooking Time: 15 minutes

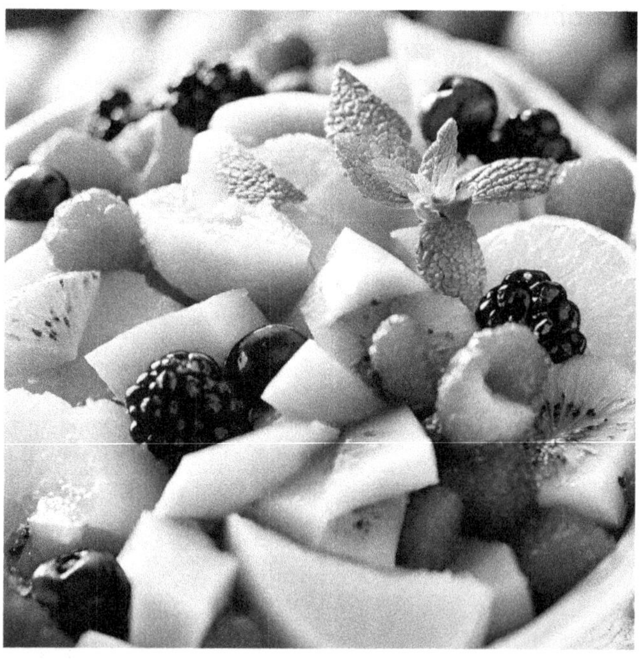

10. Apple Crisp with Oat Topping

Ingredients:

- 4 cups apples, peeled, cored, and sliced
- 1/4 cup honey
- 1 teaspoon ground cinnamon
- 1 teaspoon lemon juice
- 1 cup rolled oats
- 1/2 cup whole wheat flour
- 1/2 cup chopped walnuts
- 1/4 cup melted coconut oil
- 1/4 cup honey

Instructions:

1. Preheat the oven to 350°F (175°C).
2. In a large bowl, mix the apple slices with 1/4 cup honey, ground cinnamon, and lemon juice. Transfer to a greased 9x9-inch baking dish.
3. In another bowl, combine rolled oats, whole wheat flour, chopped walnuts, melted coconut oil, and 1/4 cup honey. Mix well.
4. Sprinkle the oat mixture over the apples.
5. Bake for 35-40 minutes, or until the topping is golden brown and the apples are tender.
6. Serve warm.

Nutrition Info (per serving):

- Calories: 220
- Protein: 3g
- Carbohydrates: 34g
- Fiber: 5g
- Sugars: 18g
- Fat: 10g
- Sodium: 5mg

Number of Servings: 6

Cooking Time: 40 minutes

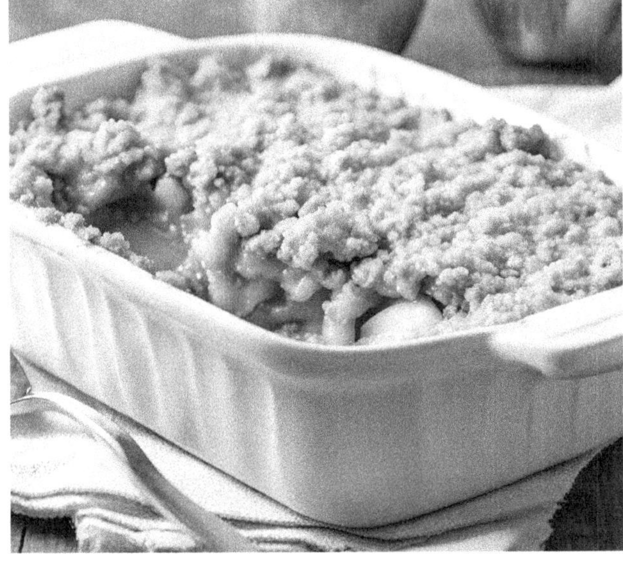

11. Strawberry Rhubarb Crumble

Ingredients:

- 2 cups strawberries, hulled and sliced
- 2 cups rhubarb, chopped
- 1/4 cup honey
- 1 teaspoon vanilla extract
- 1 cup rolled oats
- 1/2 cup whole wheat flour
- 1/4 cup coconut sugar
- 1/2 cup melted coconut oil

Instructions:

1. Preheat the oven to 350°F (175°C).
2. In a large bowl, mix strawberries, rhubarb, honey, and vanilla extract. Transfer to a greased 9x9-inch baking dish.
3. In another bowl, combine rolled oats, whole wheat flour, coconut sugar, and melted coconut oil. Mix well.
4. Sprinkle the oat mixture over the strawberry-rhubarb mixture.
5. Bake for 35-40 minutes, or until the topping is golden brown and the fruit is bubbly.
6. Serve warm.

Nutrition Info (per serving):

- Calories: 210
- Protein: 3g
- Carbohydrates: 30g
- Fiber: 4g
- Sugars: 15g
- Fat: 10g
- Sodium: 5mg

Number of Servings: 6
Cooking Time: 40 minutes

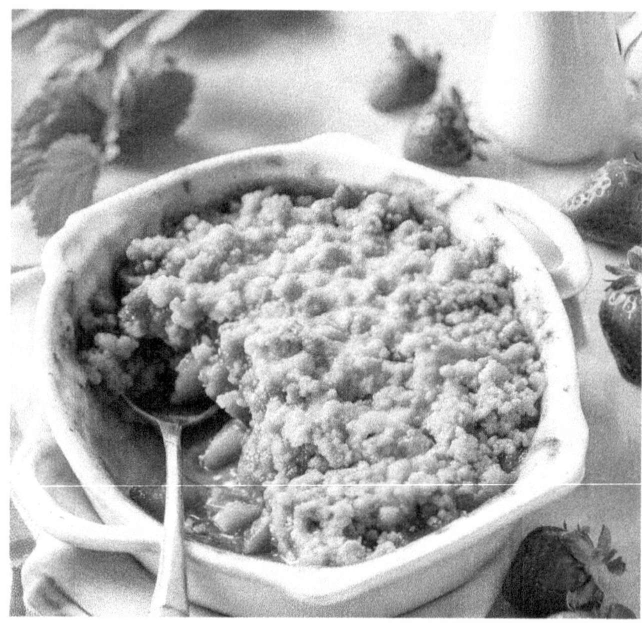

12. Fig and Almond Cake

Ingredients:

- 1 cup dried figs, chopped
- 1/2 cup almonds, ground
- 1/2 cup whole wheat flour
- 1/2 teaspoon baking powder
- 1/2 teaspoon ground cinnamon
- 1/4 teaspoon ground nutmeg
- 3 eggs
- 1/2 cup honey
- 1/2 cup Greek yogurt
- 1 teaspoon vanilla extract

Instructions:

1. Preheat the oven to 350°F (175°C). Grease a 9-inch round cake pan.
2. In a large bowl, mix ground almonds, whole wheat flour, baking powder, ground cinnamon, and ground nutmeg.
3. In another bowl, whisk eggs, honey, Greek yogurt, and vanilla extract until well combined.
4. Add the wet ingredients to the dry ingredients and mix until just combined.
5. Fold in the chopped figs.
6. Pour the batter into the prepared cake pan.
7. Bake for 30-35 minutes, or until a toothpick inserted into the center comes out clean.
8. Let cool before serving.

Nutrition Info (per serving):

- Calories: 220
- Protein: 5g
- Carbohydrates: 30g
- Fiber: 4g
- Sugars: 20g
- Fat: 10g
- Sodium: 40mg

Number of Servings: 8
Cooking Time: 35 minutes

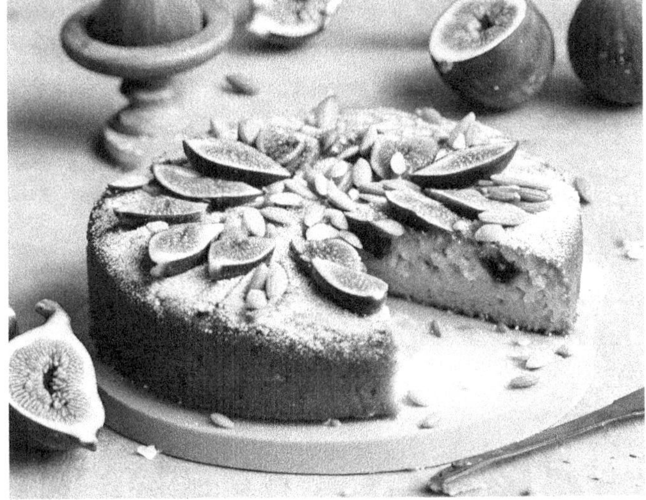

13. Whole Grain Lemon Poppy Seed Cake

Ingredients:

- 1 1/2 cups whole wheat flour
- 1/2 cup rolled oats
- 1 teaspoon baking powder
- 1/2 teaspoon baking soda
- 2 tablespoons poppy seeds
- 1/2 cup coconut oil, melted
- 1/2 cup honey
- 2 eggs
- 1/2 cup Greek yogurt
- 1/4 cup lemon juice
- 1 tablespoon lemon zest

Instructions:

1. Preheat the oven to 350°F (175°C). Grease a 9x5-inch loaf pan.
2. In a large bowl, mix whole wheat flour, rolled oats, baking powder, baking soda, and poppy seeds.
3. In another bowl, whisk melted coconut oil, honey, eggs, Greek yogurt, lemon juice, and lemon zest until well combined.
4. Add the wet ingredients to the dry ingredients and mix until just combined.
5. Pour the batter into the prepared loaf pan.
6. Bake for 40-45 minutes, or until a toothpick inserted into the center comes out clean.
7. Let cool in the pan for 10 minutes before transferring to a wire rack to cool completely.

Nutrition Info (per serving):

- Calories: 250
- Protein: 6g
- Carbohydrates: 35g
- Fiber: 4g
- Sugars: 15g
- Fat: 10g
- Sodium: 60mg

Number of Servings: 10

Cooking Time: 45 minutes

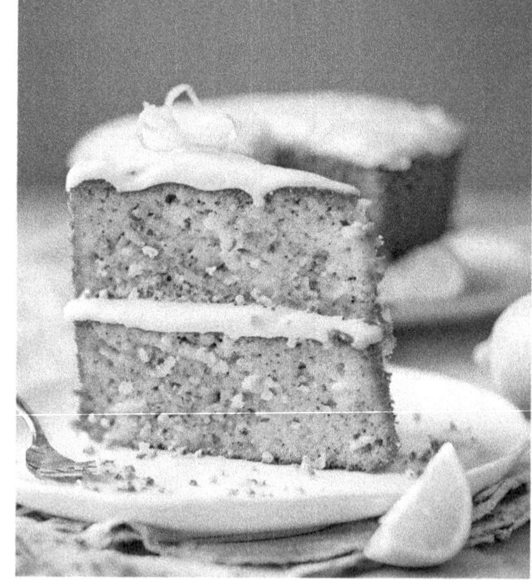

14. Ginger Pear Bread

Ingredients:

- 2 cups whole wheat flour
- 1 teaspoon baking powder
- 1/2 teaspoon baking soda
- 1 teaspoon ground ginger
- 1/2 teaspoon ground cinnamon
- 1/4 teaspoon ground nutmeg
- 1/2 cup coconut oil, melted
- 1/2 cup honey
- 2 eggs
- 1/2 cup Greek yogurt
- 1 teaspoon vanilla extract
- 2 pears, peeled and diced

Instructions:

1. Preheat the oven to 350°F (175°C). Grease a 9x5-inch loaf pan.
2. In a large bowl, mix whole wheat flour, baking powder, baking soda, ground ginger, ground cinnamon, and ground nutmeg.
3. In another bowl, whisk melted coconut oil, honey, eggs, Greek yogurt, and vanilla extract until well combined.
4. Add the wet ingredients to the dry ingredients and mix until just combined.
5. Fold in the diced pears.
6. Pour the batter into the prepared loaf pan.
7. Bake for 50-55 minutes, or until a toothpick inserted into the center comes out clean.
8. Let cool in the pan for 10 minutes before transferring to a wire rack to cool completely.

Nutrition Info (per serving):

- Calories: 200
- Protein: 4g
- Carbohydrates: 30g
- Fiber: 4g
- Sugars: 15g
- Fat: 8g
- Sodium: 70mg

Number of Servings: 10
Cooking Time: 55 minutes

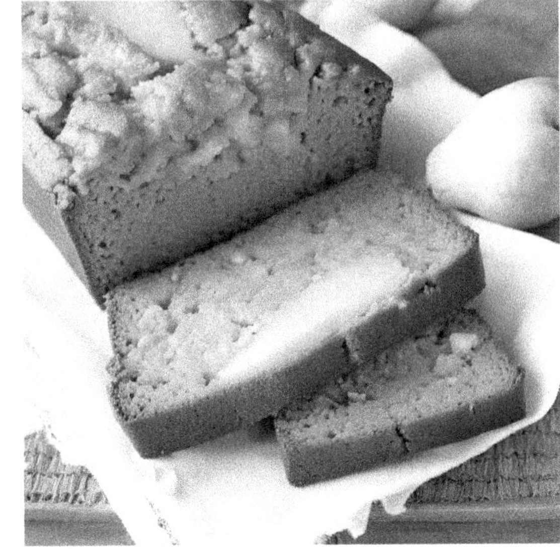

15. Walnut Stuffed Figs

Ingredients:

- 12 dried figs
- 1/4 cup walnuts, chopped
- 1 tablespoon honey
- 1/4 teaspoon ground cinnamon

Instructions:

1. Preheat the oven to 350°F (175°C).
2. Make a small slit in each fig and stuff with chopped walnuts.
3. Place the stuffed figs in a baking dish.
4. Drizzle with honey and sprinkle with ground cinnamon.
5. Bake for 10-15 minutes, or until the figs are heated through.
6. Serve warm.

Nutrition Info (per serving):

- Calories: 100
- Protein: 1g
- Carbohydrates: 18g
- Fiber: 2g
- Sugars: 14g
- Fat: 3g
- Sodium: 5mg

Number of Servings: 12

Cooking Time: 15 minutes

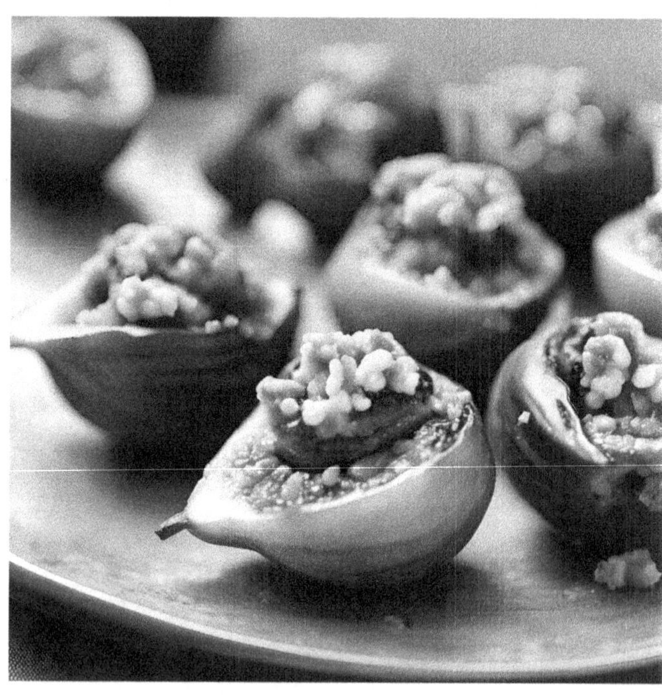

16. Spiced Baked Quinces

Ingredients:

- 4 quinces, peeled, cored, and sliced
- 1/4 cup honey
- 1 teaspoon ground cinnamon
- 1/2 teaspoon ground nutmeg
- 1/4 teaspoon ground cloves
- 1/4 cup orange juice

Instructions:

1. Preheat the oven to 350°F (175°C). Grease a baking dish.
2. Arrange the quince slices in the baking dish.
3. Drizzle with honey and sprinkle with ground cinnamon, ground nutmeg, and ground cloves.
4. Pour orange juice over the quinces.
5. Bake for 45-50 minutes, or until the quinces are tender.
6. Serve warm.

Nutrition Info (per serving):

- Calories: 100
- Protein: 0g
- Carbohydrates: 26g
- Fiber: 4g
- Sugars: 20g
- Fat: 0g
- Sodium: 5mg

Number of Servings: 8
Cooking Time: 50 minutes

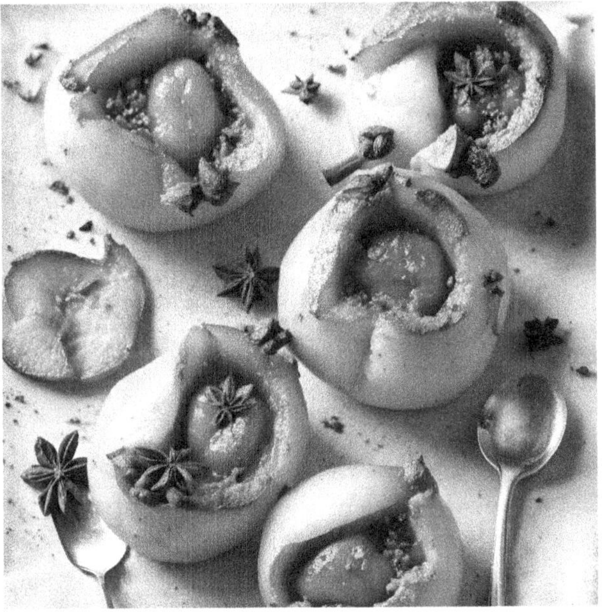

17. Pumpkin Flaxseed Muffins

Ingredients:

- 1 1/2 cups whole wheat flour
- 1/2 cup ground flaxseed
- 1 teaspoon baking powder
- 1/2 teaspoon baking soda
- 1 teaspoon ground cinnamon
- 1/2 teaspoon ground nutmeg
- 1/2 teaspoon ground ginger
- 1/4 teaspoon ground cloves
- 1/2 cup honey
- 1 cup pumpkin puree
- 1/2 cup almond milk
- 1/4 cup coconut oil, melted
- 1 teaspoon vanilla extract
- 2 large eggs

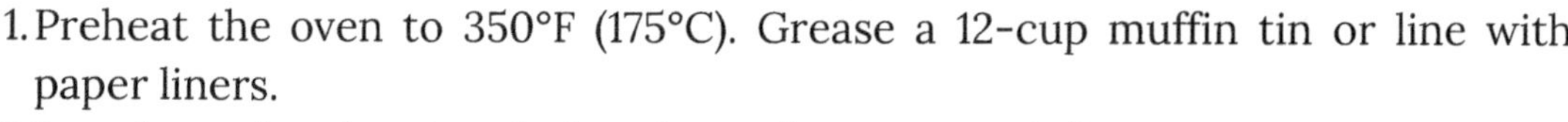

Instructions:

1. Preheat the oven to 350°F (175°C). Grease a 12-cup muffin tin or line with paper liners.
2. In a large bowl, mix whole wheat flour, ground flaxseed, baking powder, baking soda, ground cinnamon, ground nutmeg, ground ginger, and ground cloves.
3. In another bowl, whisk honey, pumpkin puree, almond milk, melted coconut oil, vanilla extract, and eggs until well combined.
4. Add the wet ingredients to the dry ingredients and stir until just combined.
5. Divide the batter evenly among the muffin cups.
6. Bake for 20-25 minutes, or until a toothpick inserted into the center comes out clean.
7. Let cool for a few minutes before serving.

Nutrition Info (per serving):

- Calories: 180
- Protein: 4g
- Carbohydrates: 26g
- Fiber: 4g
- Sugars: 12g
- Fat: 7g
- Sodium: 70mg

Number of Servings: 12
Cooking Time: 25 minutes

18. Cranberry Orange Nut Bread

Ingredients:

- 2 cups whole wheat flour
- 1/2 cup coconut sugar
- 1 teaspoon baking powder
- 1/2 teaspoon baking soda
- 1/2 teaspoon ground cinnamon
- 1/4 teaspoon ground nutmeg
- 1/2 cup fresh orange juice
- 1/4 cup coconut oil, melted
- 1 teaspoon vanilla extract
- 2 large eggs
- 1 cup fresh cranberries
- 1/2 cup chopped walnuts
- 1 tablespoon orange zest

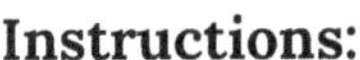

Instructions:

1. Preheat the oven to 350°F (175°C). Grease a 9x5-inch loaf pan.
2. In a large bowl, mix whole wheat flour, coconut sugar, baking powder, baking soda, ground cinnamon, and ground nutmeg.
3. In another bowl, whisk fresh orange juice, melted coconut oil, vanilla extract, and eggs until well combined.
4. Add the wet ingredients to the dry ingredients and stir until just combined.
5. Fold in the fresh cranberries, chopped walnuts, and orange zest.
6. Pour the batter into the prepared loaf pan.
7. Bake for 50-55 minutes, or until a toothpick inserted into the center comes out clean.
8. Let cool in the pan for 10 minutes before transferring to a wire rack to cool completely.

Nutrition Info (per serving):

- Calories: 200
- Protein: 4g
- Carbohydrates: 30g
- Fiber: 4g
- Sugars: 15g
- Fat: 8g
- Sodium: 70mg

Number of Servings: 10

Cooking Time: 55 minutes

9-WEEK MEAL PLAN

Week 1
Monday
- **Breakfast:** Apple Cinnamon Baked Oatmeal Cups
- **Lunch:** Grilled Chicken Salad with Mixed Greens
- **Dinner:** Slow-Cooked Beef Stew
- **Snack:** Walnut Stuffed Figs

Tuesday
- **Breakfast:** Banana Nut Bread
- **Lunch:** Shrimp and Spinach Salad
- **Dinner:** Grilled Sirloin Steak
- **Snack:** Almond and Date Truffles

Wednesday
- **Breakfast:** Chia Seed Pudding with Berries
- **Lunch:** Turkey and Spinach Stuffed Peppers
- **Dinner:** Pork and Apple Stew
- **Snack:** Fruit Salad with Citrus Mint Dressing

Thursday
- **Breakfast:** Whole Grain Blueberry Muffins
- **Lunch:** Balsamic Glazed Chicken Breasts
- **Dinner:** Beef and Broccoli Stir-Fry
- **Snack:** Cranberry Orange Nut Bread

Friday
- **Breakfast:** Baked Pears with Honey and Walnuts
- **Lunch:** Chicken Noodle Soup
- **Dinner:** Balsamic Glazed Beef Roast
- **Snack:** No-Bake Chocolate Oat Bars

Saturday
- **Breakfast:** Carrot Cake with Cream Cheese Frosting
- **Lunch:** Chicken Caesar Wrap
- **Dinner:** Grilled Pork Tenderloin
- **Snack:** Apricot and Seed Bars

Sunday
- **Breakfast:** Whole Grain Lemon Poppy Seed Cake
- **Lunch:** Chicken and Vegetable Stir-Fry
- **Dinner:** Pork Chops with Peach Salsa
- **Snack:** Spiced Baked Quinces

Week 2

Monday
- **Breakfast:** Ginger Pear Bread
- **Lunch:** Beef Barley Soup
- **Dinner:** Thai Beef Salad
- **Snack:** Apple Crisp with Oat Topping

Tuesday
- **Breakfast:** Pumpkin Flaxseed Muffins
- **Lunch:** Greek Chicken Skewers
- **Dinner:** Beef Goulash
- **Snack:** Almond and Date Truffles

Wednesday
- **Breakfast:** Carrot Cake with Cream Cheese Frosting
- **Lunch:** Chicken Piccata
- **Dinner:** Pork Miso Soup
- **Snack:** Walnut Stuffed Figs

Thursday
- **Breakfast:** Baked Pears with Honey and Walnuts
- **Lunch:** Italian Beef Ragu
- **Dinner:** Chicken Tabbouleh Salad
- **Snack:** Fruit Salad with Citrus Mint Dressing

Friday
- **Breakfast:** Whole Grain Blueberry Muffins
- **Lunch:** Smoked Turkey Breast on Rye
- **Dinner:** Swedish Meatballs
- **Snack:** No-Bake Chocolate Oat Bars

Saturday
- **Breakfast:** Chia Seed Pudding with Berries
- **Lunch:** Chicken Vegetable Pot Pie
- **Dinner:** Beef and Mushroom Skillet
- **Snack:** Cranberry Orange Nut Bread

Sunday
- **Breakfast:** Apple Cinnamon Baked Oatmeal Cups
- **Lunch:** Asian Turkey Lettuce Wraps
- **Dinner:** Pulled Pork with BBQ Sauce
- **Snack:** Apricot and Seed Bars

Week 3

Monday
- **Breakfast:** Banana Nut Bread
- **Lunch:** Grilled Chicken and Pineapple Skewers
- **Dinner:** Beef Goulash
- **Snack:** Almond and Date Truffles

Tuesday
- **Breakfast:** Pumpkin Flaxseed Muffins
- **Lunch:** Beef Carpaccio
- **Dinner:** Moroccan Chicken with Couscous
- **Snack:** Fruit Salad with Citrus Mint Dressing

Wednesday
- **Breakfast:** Ginger Pear Bread
- **Lunch:** Pork and Pepper Stir-Fry
- **Dinner:** Chicken and Barley Soup
- **Snack:** Apple Crisp with Oat Topping

Thursday
- **Breakfast:** Whole Grain Lemon Poppy Seed Cake
- **Lunch:** Vietnamese Pork Bowls
- **Dinner:** Balsamic Glazed Beef Roast
- **Snack:** Spiced Baked Quinces

Friday
- **Breakfast:** Chia Seed Pudding with Berries
- **Lunch:** Chicken Fajitas
- **Dinner:** Slow Cooker Chicken and Lentils
- **Snack:** Cranberry Orange Nut Bread

Saturday
- **Breakfast:** Apple Cinnamon Baked Oatmeal Cups
- **Lunch:** Pork Loin Roast with Herbs
- **Dinner:** Chicken and Spinach Quiche
- **Snack:** No-Bake Chocolate Oat Bars

Sunday
- **Breakfast:** Whole Grain Blueberry Muffins
- **Lunch:** Chicken Noodle Soup
- **Dinner:** Pork Miso Soup
- **Snack:** Walnut Stuffed Figs

Week 4

Monday
- **Breakfast:** Baked Pears with Honey and Walnuts
- **Lunch:** Grilled Pork Tenderloin
- **Dinner:** Beef and Broccoli Stir-Fry
- **Snack:** Almond and Date Truffles

Tuesday
- **Breakfast:** Pumpkin Flaxseed Muffins
- **Lunch:** Chicken Caesar Wrap
- **Dinner:** Grilled Sirloin Steak
- **Snack:** Apple Crisp with Oat Topping

Wednesday
- **Breakfast:** Banana Nut Bread
- **Lunch:** Thai Beef Salad
- **Dinner:** Pork and Apple Stew
- **Snack:** Fruit Salad with Citrus Mint Dressing

Thursday
- **Breakfast:** Ginger Pear Bread
- **Lunch:** Turkey Meatballs in Tomato Sauce
- **Dinner:** Moroccan Chicken with Couscous
- **Snack:** Cranberry Orange Nut Bread

Friday
- **Breakfast:** Whole Grain Lemon Poppy Seed Cake
- **Lunch:** Chicken Vegetable Pot Pie
- **Dinner:** Balsamic Glazed Chicken Breasts
- **Snack:** No-Bake Chocolate Oat Bars

Saturday
- **Breakfast:** Chia Seed Pudding with Berries
- **Lunch:** Swedish Meatballs
- **Dinner:** Beef Goulash
- **Snack:** Walnut Stuffed Figs

Sunday
- **Breakfast:** Whole Grain Blueberry Muffins
- **Lunch:** Chicken and Spinach Quiche
- **Dinner:** Pulled Pork with BBQ Sauce
- **Snack:** Apricot and Seed Bars

Week 5

Monday
- **Breakfast:** Apple Cinnamon Baked Oatmeal Cups
- **Lunch:** Chicken Tabbouleh Salad
- **Dinner:** Slow-Cooked Beef Stew
- **Snack:** Walnut Stuffed Figs

Tuesday
- **Breakfast:** Banana Nut Bread
- **Lunch:** Beef and Mushroom Skillet
- **Dinner:** Grilled Sirloin Steak
- **Snack:** Almond and Date Truffles

Wednesday
- **Breakfast:** Chia Seed Pudding with Berries
- **Lunch:** Grilled Chicken Salad with Mixed Greens
- **Dinner:** Pork and Pepper Stir-Fry
- **Snack:** Fruit Salad with Citrus Mint Dressing

Thursday
- **Breakfast:** Whole Grain Blueberry Muffins
- **Lunch:** Chicken Caesar Wrap
- **Dinner:** Balsamic Glazed Beef Roast
- **Snack:** Cranberry Orange Nut Bread

Friday
- **Breakfast:** Baked Pears with Honey and Walnuts
- **Lunch:** Thai Beef Salad
- **Dinner:** Italian Beef Ragu
- **Snack:** No-Bake Chocolate Oat Bars

Saturday
- **Breakfast:** Carrot Cake with Cream Cheese Frosting
- **Lunch:** Chicken Fajitas
- **Dinner:** Pulled Pork with BBQ Sauce
- **Snack:** Apricot and Seed Bars

Sunday
- **Breakfast:** Whole Grain Lemon Poppy Seed Cake
- **Lunch:** Greek Chicken Skewers
- **Dinner:** Beef Goulash
- **Snack:** Spiced Baked Quinces

Week 6

Monday
- **Breakfast:** Ginger Pear Bread
- **Lunch:** Chicken and Spinach Quiche
- **Dinner:** Beef Barley Soup
- **Snack:** Apple Crisp with Oat Topping

Tuesday
- **Breakfast:** Pumpkin Flaxseed Muffins
- **Lunch:** Swedish Meatballs
- **Dinner:** Moroccan Chicken with Couscous
- **Snack:** Almond and Date Truffles

Wednesday
- **Breakfast:** Carrot Cake with Cream Cheese Frosting
- **Lunch:** Turkey Meatballs in Tomato Sauce
- **Dinner:** Chicken Piccata
- **Snack:** Walnut Stuffed Figs

Thursday
- **Breakfast:** Baked Pears with Honey and Walnuts
- **Lunch:** Vietnamese Pork Bowls
- **Dinner:** Chicken and Barley Soup
- **Snack:** Fruit Salad with Citrus Mint Dressing

Friday
- **Breakfast:** Whole Grain Blueberry Muffins
- **Lunch:** Beef Carpaccio
- **Dinner:** Grilled Pork Tenderloin
- **Snack:** No-Bake Chocolate Oat Bars

Saturday
- **Breakfast:** Chia Seed Pudding with Berries
- **Lunch:** Chicken Vegetable Pot Pie
- **Dinner:** Grilled Chicken and Pineapple Skewers
- **Snack:** Cranberry Orange Nut Bread

Sunday
- **Breakfast:** Apple Cinnamon Baked Oatmeal Cups
- **Lunch:** Chicken Noodle Soup
- **Dinner:** Pork Miso Soup
- **Snack:** Apricot and Seed Bars

Week 7

Monday
- **Breakfast:** Banana Nut Bread
- **Lunch:** Chicken and Vegetable Stir-Fry
- **Dinner:** Pork and Apple Stew
- **Snack:** Almond and Date Truffles

Tuesday
- **Breakfast:** Pumpkin Flaxseed Muffins
- **Lunch:** Asian Turkey Lettuce Wraps
- **Dinner:** Beef and Broccoli Stir-Fry
- **Snack:** Fruit Salad with Citrus Mint Dressing

Wednesday
- **Breakfast:** Ginger Pear Bread
- **Lunch:** Slow Cooker Chicken and Lentils
- **Dinner:** Balsamic Glazed Beef Roast
- **Snack:** Apple Crisp with Oat Topping

Thursday
- **Breakfast:** Whole Grain Lemon Poppy Seed Cake
- **Lunch:** Chicken Caesar Wrap
- **Dinner:** Beef Goulash
- **Snack:** Spiced Baked Quinces

Friday
- **Breakfast:** Chia Seed Pudding with Berries
- **Lunch:** Pulled Pork with BBQ Sauce
- **Dinner:** Pork Loin Roast with Herbs
- **Snack:** Cranberry Orange Nut Bread

Saturday
- **Breakfast:** Apple Cinnamon Baked Oatmeal Cups
- **Lunch:** Chicken Tabbouleh Salad
- **Dinner:** Moroccan Chicken with Couscous
- **Snack:** No-Bake Chocolate Oat Bars

Sunday
- **Breakfast:** Whole Grain Blueberry Muffins
- **Lunch:** Beef and Mushroom Skillet
- **Dinner:** Beef Barley Soup
- **Snack:** Walnut Stuffed Figs

Week 8

Monday
- **Breakfast:** Baked Pears with Honey and Walnuts
- **Lunch:** Chicken Piccata
- **Dinner:** Pork and Pepper Stir-Fry
- **Snack:** Almond and Date Truffles

Tuesday
- **Breakfast:** Pumpkin Flaxseed Muffins
- **Lunch:** Beef Carpaccio
- **Dinner:** Grilled Sirloin Steak
- **Snack:** Apple Crisp with Oat Topping

Wednesday
- **Breakfast:** Banana Nut Bread
- **Lunch:** Grilled Pork Tenderloin
- **Dinner:** Chicken and Barley Soup
- **Snack:** Fruit Salad with Citrus Mint Dressing

Thursday
- **Breakfast:** Ginger Pear Bread
- **Lunch:** Thai Beef Salad
- **Dinner:** Italian Beef Ragu
- **Snack:** Cranberry Orange Nut Bread

Friday
- **Breakfast:** Whole Grain Lemon Poppy Seed Cake
- **Lunch:** Chicken and Vegetable Stir-Fry
- **Dinner:** Grilled Chicken and Pineapple Skewers
- **Snack:** No-Bake Chocolate Oat Bars

Saturday
- **Breakfast:** Chia Seed Pudding with Berries
- **Lunch:** Beef Goulash
- **Dinner:** Beef and Broccoli Stir-Fry
- **Snack:** Walnut Stuffed Figs

Sunday
- **Breakfast:** Whole Grain Blueberry Muffins
- **Lunch:** Moroccan Chicken with Couscous
- **Dinner:** Pork Miso Soup
- **Snack:** Apricot and Seed Bars

Week 9

Monday
- **Breakfast:** Apple Cinnamon Baked Oatmeal Cups
- **Lunch:** Chicken Caesar Wrap
- **Dinner:** Slow-Cooked Beef Stew
- **Snack:** Walnut Stuffed Figs

Tuesday
- **Breakfast:** Banana Nut Bread
- **Lunch:** Greek Chicken Skewers
- **Dinner:** Grilled Sirloin Steak
- **Snack:** Almond and Date Truffles

Wednesday
- **Breakfast:** Chia Seed Pudding with Berries
- **Lunch:** Chicken Noodle Soup
- **Dinner:** Pork and Apple Stew
- **Snack:** Fruit Salad with Citrus Mint Dressing

Thursday
- **Breakfast:** Whole Grain Blueberry Muffins
- **Lunch:** Asian Turkey Lettuce Wraps
- **Dinner:** Balsamic Glazed Beef Roast
- **Snack:** Cranberry Orange Nut Bread

Friday
- **Breakfast:** Baked Pears with Honey and Walnuts
- **Lunch:** Chicken Tabbouleh Salad
- **Dinner:** Beef and Mushroom Skillet
- **Snack:** No-Bake Chocolate Oat Bars

Saturday
- **Breakfast:** Carrot Cake with Cream Cheese Frosting
- **Lunch:** Pulled Pork with BBQ Sauce
- **Dinner:** Grilled Pork Tenderloin
- **Snack:** Apricot and Seed Bars

Sunday
- **Breakfast:** Whole Grain Lemon Poppy Seed Cake
- **Lunch:** Chicken Piccata
- **Dinner:** Pork Miso Soup
- **Snack:** Spiced Baked Quinces

WEEKLY MEAL PLANNER JOURNAL

	BREAKFAST	LUNCH	DINNER	SNACKS
MON				
TUE				
WED				
THU				
FRI				
SAT				
SUN				

What are your primary health goals for following the COPD diet? How do you believe this diet will help improve your condition?

WEEKLY MEAL PLANNER JOURNAL

	BREAKFAST	LUNCH	DINNER	SNACKS
MON				
TUE				
WED				
THU				
FRI				
SAT				
SUN				

What specific aspects of the COPD diet do you find most challenging to understand?
How can you seek clarification on these points?

WEEKLY MEAL PLANNER JOURNAL

	BREAKFAST	LUNCH	DINNER	SNACKS
MON				
TUE				
WED				
THU				
FRI				
SAT				
SUN				

Describe your current eating habits. What are the main changes you anticipate making when you switch to the COPD diet?

WEEKLY MEAL PLANNER JOURNAL

	BREAKFAST	LUNCH	DINNER	SNACKS
MON				
TUE				
WED				
THU				
FRI				
SAT				
SUN				

How will you adjust your grocery shopping list to align with the COPD diet? What new foods will you add, and which will you reduce or eliminate?

WEEKLY MEAL PLANNER JOURNAL

	BREAKFAST	LUNCH	DINNER	SNACKS
MON				
TUE				
WED				
THU				
FRI				
SAT				
SUN				

Which COPD-friendly recipes are you most excited to try? Why do these recipes appeal to you?

WEEKLY MEAL PLANNER JOURNAL

	BREAKFAST	LUNCH	DINNER	SNACKS
MON				
TUE				
WED				
THU				
FRI				
SAT				
SUN				

What are your specific nutritional needs as a COPD patient? How does the COPD diet address these needs?

WEEKLY MEAL PLANNER JOURNAL

	BREAKFAST	LUNCH	DINNER	SNACKS
MON				
TUE				
WED				
THU				
FRI				
SAT				
SUN				

How do you plan to stick to the COPD diet when eating out at restaurants or social gatherings? What are some strategies you can use?

WEEKLY MEAL PLANNER JOURNAL

	BREAKFAST	LUNCH	DINNER	SNACKS
MON				
TUE				
WED				
THU				
FRI				
SAT				
SUN				

Who in your life can support you as you transition to the COPD diet? How can they help you stay motivated and on track?

WEEKLY MEAL PLANNER JOURNAL

	BREAKFAST	LUNCH	DINNER	SNACKS
MON				
TUE				
WED				
THU				
FRI				
SAT				
SUN				

What potential challenges do you foresee when starting the COPD diet? What solutions or strategies can you prepare in advance to overcome these challenges?

Scan the QR code below to get a surprise bonus!

www.ingramcontent.com/pod-product-compliance
Lightning Source LLC
Chambersburg PA
CBHW081213260726
48653CB00010BA/3636